MW00474627

"... a very practical text offering insights and techniques that can be directly applied to clinical work with real patients. This book explores the theory of chakra healing, offering ideas about mind-body medicine and the subtle energies sensed by the practitioner and patient alike."

–Val Hopwood, PhD, MSc, FCSP, *Journal of the Acupuncture Association of Chartered Physiotherapists*

"Overall, this is a most interesting and inspiring book that describes the use of chakra balancing in the healing process in a very readable and accessible manner."

–Linda J. Skellam, MCSP, *Association of Chartered Physiotherapists in Reflextherapy Newsletter*

"John Cross explores the many themes with his unique mixture of delicacy and robust humor. The whole book induces a pleasant sense of having entered a world of a considerably talented clinician and teacher."

–Pam Elstub, MCSP, *Association of Chartered Physiotherapists in Energy Medicine Newsletter*

ACUPUNCTURE AND THE CHAKRA ENERGY SYSTEM

Treating the *Cause* of Disease

JOHN R. CROSS

FCSP, DrAc, SRP; MRSH

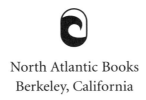

North Atlantic Books
Berkeley, California

Published by
North Atlantic Books
P.O. Box 12327
Berkeley, California 94712

Cover and book design
© Ayelet Maida, A/M Studios

Cover art © Ayelet Maida; yinyang source art © John Woodcock, iStock.com
Illustrations © 2008 Donald and Pam Budge, Croft Studio Dunvegan, Isle of Skye, Scotland.

Permissions
Figure 1.4 (Associations of the Major Chakras with the Autonomic Nervous System) reproduced from Gray's Anatomy by Donald and Pam Budge of Croft Studio with kind permission from Lippincott Williams and Wilkins.

Printed in the United States of America

Acupuncture and the Chakra Energy System: Treating the Cause *of Disease* is sponsored by the Society for the Study of Native Arts and Sciences, a nonprofit educational corporation whose goals are to develop an educational and cross-cultural perspective linking various scientific, social, and artistic fields; to nurture a holistic view of arts, sciences, humanities, and healing; and to publish and distribute literature on the relationship of mind, body, and nature.

North Atlantic Books' publications are available through most bookstores. For further information, call 800-733-3000 or visit our Web site at www.northatlanticbooks.com.

MEDICAL DISCLAIMER: The following information is intended for general information purposes only. Individuals should always see their health care provider before administering any suggestions made in this book. Any application of the material set forth in the following pages is at the reader's discretion and is his or her sole responsibility.

Library of Congress Cataloging-in-Publication Data

Cross, John R., Dr.
    Acupuncture and the chakra energy system : treating the cause of disease / John R. Cross.
        p. ; cm.
    Includes bibliographical references and index.
    Summary: "A sequel to *Healing with the Chakra Energy System,* this book combines traditional Chinese acupuncture analysis and treatment with the chakra energy system of Ayurvedic philosophy"—Provided by publisher.
    ISBN 978-1-55643-721-2
    1. Acupuncture. 2. Chakras. 3. Medicine, Chinese. 4. Medicine, Ayurvedic. I. Title.
    [DNLM: 1. Acupuncture Therapy—methods. 2. Medicine, Ayurvedic. 3. Medicine, Chinese Traditional. 4. Mind-Body and Relaxation Techniques. WB 369 C951a 2008]
    RM184.C76 2008
    615.8'92—dc22   2008007217

2 3 4 5 6 7 8 9 SHERIDAN 14 13 12 11 10 09

This book is dedicated to my children Bethany and Toby, who along with my grandchildren Jack, Ben, and Louisa have been responsible for keeping my feet "on the ground."

Bless you!

CONTENTS

Chapter One

THE CHAKRAS — 1

Chapter Two

TRADITIONAL CHINESE MEDICINE AND THE CHAKRAS — 51

Chapter Three

TREATMENT OF PAIN — 89

Chapter Four

TREATMENT OF CHRONIC CONDITIONS — 115

LIST OF ILLUSTRATIONS

FOREWORD

It is an honor and privilege to write the foreword for this book. I was first made aware of the existence of the chakras in relation to acupuncture at one of John's excellent seminars for physiotherapists. The challenges faced by practitioners to improve the efficacy of treatments and to explore the underlying reasons for successful outcomes are infinite. This book addresses the theory and practice of acupuncture and relates acupuncture points with the sites of the chakras, an important concept in Ayurvedic medicine. This in itself has been a breakthrough in finding the connection between two different traditional medicine concepts. John has further addressed this basic relationship to include a comprehensive system of diagnosis and treatment. This approach has influenced a great number of therapists, including myself, who have found their practice enhanced by using these techniques.

This book does not offer a large reference of controlled trials; however, it gives the reader the opportunity to learn from John's vast clinical experience. The knowledge it contains is invaluable and demonstrates how the manipulation of subtle energies of the body can contribute toward successful treatments. John comprehensively writes of the many similarities and differences in chakra energy and acupuncture theory. In the following pages there is much to take "on board." The journey, though, will be very worthwhile.

Nadia Ellis MSc, FCSP, LicAc
Past president of the Acupuncture Association
of Chartered Physiotherapists and author of
*Acupuncture in Clinical Practice: A Guide for
Health Professionals* (Chapman and Hall, 1994)

FOREWORD

I have never met Dr. John Cross. However, that does not mean I do not know him. Having been an avid reader of his three previous publications, *Healing with the Chakra Energy System, Acupressure and Reflextherapy in the Treatment of Medical Conditions,* and *Acupressure Clinical Applications in Musculo-Skeletal Conditions,* I have been able to get into his head and his spirit and feel as though I know him well. I have spent days and weeks with Dr. Cross through the pages of his academic works. We have been to the beach, cruised the Mediterranean, flown to Germany as well as Australia, and even met by flashlight in a tent on the rim of the Grand Canyon. I have digested, read, and re-read all three previous publications a multitude of times. I can truly say I know Dr. John Cross.

When he asked me if I would write the foreword to his latest book *Acupuncture and the Chakra Energy System,* I was both honored and humbled beyond description. Even though I reside in Arizona and John lives in the Isle of Skye in Scotland and our worlds are eons apart as to culture and environment, however, we are both doctors and healers and share an undying interest in the chakra system of the body and how it affects human health. John had happened to read several articles I had written concerning the chakra system of the body and realized that we had a great deal in common. For this reason, he asked if I would write his foreword.

Having been an educator of acupuncture since 1977 and a practitioner of acupuncture since 1971, my education, lectures, and travels have taken me to virtually all corners of the globe. In the mid-seventies while in a remote area of Southeast Asia I was introduced to the chakra system of the body. That chance encounter with the chakra system led me on a quest to learn what was available worldwide through a variety of venues. I have encountered esoteric and extreme esoteric applications and have seen and experienced many brands of chakra application. Many had merit, but most did not.

With my background in chakras I had reached a very comfortable place in my life and practice with my knowledge of this huge topic. As a practitioner of acupuncture I combined these two healing arts and created what would become a very successful clinical practice with which a multitude of conditions were successfully treated.

When I learned Dr. Cross was in the planning stages of *Acupuncture and the Chakra Energy System,* I was naturally excited as this book would focus on my expertise in healing, the chakras, and acupuncture. I was very familiar with this topic, and I was interested to see what he would say.

When I received the manuscript of this book to read, I was not prepared for what I was about to see. What I held in my hands was without question one of the most brilliant, academic, practical clinical essays on this topic I had ever encountered in over thirty-five years. When I stated earlier I was honored by Dr. Cross asking me to write the foreword to this book I did not realize that was just the beginning of what would be a truly humbling experience.

It was quite evident from reading this important book that Dr. Cross has not forgotten *anything* about the chakra system! *Acupuncture and the Chakra Energy System* is truly a work of gargantuan proportions.

Not only does he impart his vast knowledge of the topic of chakras, but he relays information in a way that is entertaining and light. His observations and side comments about life in general are priceless. He is truly a gifted writer, educator, and healer.

Anyone in the field of acupuncture can read and apply Dr. Cross's methods, regardless of whether they are a Traditional Chinese Medicine (TCM) practitioner, a Five Element, Korean, Japanese, European, or any other kind of practitioner. The diagrams are clear and concise, and the academic explanations do not leave anything to the imagination.

Once you begin to read this book, you will realize what you have before you. Allow Dr. John Cross to take this book from your hands, bring it to your head and your heart, and apply the healing principles. Then, all of us who read this book will be in a position to benefit mankind with clinical results and ease of application which has few—if any—equals.

John A. Amaro DC, LAc, FIAMA,
DiplAc (NCCAOM) (IAMA)
President of the International Academy
of Medical Acupuncture

INTRODUCTION

In November 2005 I approached North Atlantic books about publishing my completed manuscript, *Healing with the Chakra Energy System.* The book contained practical chapters on how to use this system of healing with acupressure, bodywork, reflexology, healing, *and* acupuncture. I had originally planned to discuss the subject of acupuncture in that book because of the enormous rise in popularity of acupuncture over the past few years and the fact that acupuncture has been regarded in many quarters as being part of mainstream medicine. The publishers informed me that the tome was too large and that they thought that two books would be better than one. That news gave me the wonderful opportunity to address the topic of acupuncture in a much more detailed manner than the original chapter had allowed me to do.

In 1987 I completed an acupuncture doctoral thesis for the British College of Acupuncture entitled "The use of Acupuncture in Relationship with the Chakra Energy System." I remember that it took over nine months to mark because it had to be read in its entirety by at least three doctors of acupuncture who were scattered around the globe and who understood what I was writing about. It is hard to imagine that this happened over twenty years ago. There was no Internet in those days and word processors were in their infancy, so it was all methodically typed out. When I look at the original thesis now, I cringe at the amateurish way it was presented.

The practice of acupuncture in the UK was very different in those days as well. For example, in 1983 when a group of physiotherapists came together to form the Acupuncture Association of Chartered Physiotherapists, there were fewer than fifty members. In 2007 this number has grown to 5,000. Going back even further, when I qualified in acupuncture (LicAc) in 1978, there were only three of us practicing acupuncture in the whole county of Devon (where I lived at the time)—I kid you not!

The proliferation of professionals who practice acupuncture has accelerated at an enormous rate—it seems that there is at least one acupuncturist in each and every city. Not only has the number of registered acupuncturists flourished over the past fifteen to twenty years, but so has the number of traditional and complementary medicine practitioners who use acupuncture as an adjunct to their main therapeutic discipline. Even ten years ago it was rare to find acupuncture being practiced in the United Kingdom's National Health Service, but now it seems commonplace to offer patients acupuncture in both situations. By contrast, in America acupuncture is still only available from private practitioners for the most part.

One of the main reasons this has taken place is that acupuncture, especially in pain relief, has been scientifically researched sufficiently as to make its practice part of mainstream medicine. This situation is to be generally applauded. There are, of course, drawbacks and snags with the continued acceptance of this apparently strange form of medicine. Sadly, there are innumerable practitioners who only attend acupuncture courses that last a couple of weekends. These people call themselves *acupuncturists* (not "registered" however) and can proceed to wreak havoc and mayhem on the gullible and unsuspecting public. With a very small knowledge base in a foreign therapeutic approach, there is little wonder that many of these practitioners become disillusioned when the treatment does not "work."

There is also a proliferation of short courses that teach one or more of the Western approaches to acupuncture. These mostly involve using this noble art as a pain relief modality with the use of "trigger" points and formulas. I have coined this type of approach "symptomatic pinpricking." It is *not* acupuncture. To practice acupuncture with any degree of confidence and depth, a student needs to have attended a course of at least two years duration. One simply cannot *just* learn one single aspect of acupuncture and omit the remainder—especially when that encompasses a wealth of knowledge of traditional approaches spanning over five thousand years.

There are, of course, many acupuncture practitioners who don't give a fig about Traditional Chinese Medicine (TCM), thinking the ideas of *chi, yin* and *yang,* meridians, Five Elements, and "energy" dated and archaic. These people, rightly or wrongly, assume that all medicine has to be scientifically-based. My personal view is that there is nothing wrong with Western scientific acupuncture, as long as the roots of our noble art are not totally forgotten. Modern scientific and research-based approaches should be mixed with traditional practices so as to give the practitioner a rounded educational and practical knowledge base. This will surely be to the benefit of both therapist and patient.

Therapy of any kind needs to be evidence-based and scientifically quantified simply because we are living in a scientific age. However, not everything can be proved scientifically. As stated before, pain relief acupuncture has been researched ad nauseum as to its physiological basis. But it is quite another thing, to obtain scientific proof of the acupuncture treatment of, say, skin conditions or non-painful organic or emotional ones. It has been shown that TCM can work wonders in these conditions, and even though its theoretical paradigms may appear quaint and out-dated, so far we do not have any other language to explain what is occurring within the deeper economy of the body.

As you may have gathered by now, I am a fan of the traditional and naturopathic approaches to therapy. One of natural medicine's principles is the belief that a high percentage of our physical and organic conditions stem from an imbalance of our emotions. This is one of the cornerstones of using the chakras with acupuncture: to create harmony from disharmony within our energetic framework and to attempt to treat the *cause* of the disease *(dis-ease),* which is often of an emotional etiology. Although TCM alone is capable of achieving this, it is *only* by focusing on the chakras that we can be certain that energy harmony has been achieved and the root cause of the condition treated.

Indeed, it was this yearning to treat the whole person—mind and body—and the desire never to suppress symptoms that led me to combine the chakra energy system and TCM. In 1985, when I was just beginning my research into this brand new method of healing, I was very much aware that the chakras had previously been best known for their use with reiki, healing, meditation, and yoga. What I have done in this book is to simplify the system by taking out the esoteric "magic" that has for so long surrounded the chakras. I would earnestly ask you, the acupuncturist of whatever persuasion, to try out the methods shown—you will find that they work!

As you may have guessed, using acupuncture with the chakra energy system does not represent a research-based approach. Almost everything in this book is original work that has taken me over twenty-five years to perfect so that I may share with you the wonders of this approach. Due to a lack of time, none of the ideas and methods described have been put to scientific scrutiny. There is, however, a huge stack of letters in my filing cabinet from grateful patients, acupuncturists, and students that offer testimony to my methods—so a huge groundswell of anecdotal appreciation is in existence. I would welcome anyone to test my conclusions in controlled trials, and I am willing to help in any way I can. Science *is* gradually proving the existence of subtle energies with which therapists work, so it should not be such a giant leap to be able to prove the efficacy of my methods. Acupuncture is a far easier modality to use in controlled trials than, say, acupressure. The latter tends to be subjective, whereas acupuncture is not.

So, how can acupuncture be used with such an esoteric system of healing? This is a question that I have heard from many quarters. Because the chakras are linked so closely with the aura and the subtle energies, many practitioners are skeptical about an approach that does not use the hands. They accept the idea of using the chakras with hands-off healing and even accept the use of contact healing that utilizes acupressure, reflexology, and cranio-sacral therapy philosophy. When it comes to sticking needles in patients and purporting to be using the chakras, however, they are rightly confused and reticent of the whole idea. The answer, my dear Watson, is simple!

As was explained in my previous book *Healing with the Chakra Energy System* and will be expounded upon in the first chapter, each major and minor chakra has a link with the physical body as an acupoint. It may be said that every acupoint on the body's surface represents a "mini" chakra. Each and every acupoint, *tsubo,* or reflex point is said to be a point of energy *(chi)* that resonates at a particular frequency. Each physical aspect of a major and minor chakra represents a particularly powerful meridian or non-meridian acupoint. This energy may be used with acupuncture as easily as with the hands. By using the acupoints of Traditional Chinese Medicine (TCM), we may influence the flow of *chi* within the body, which in turn activates the other aspects of the chakra in a more subtle way.

Just as the Etheric, Emotional, and Mental auras may influence the Physical Body, stimulation of the physical aspect of the chakras may influence the Etheric, et al. It is not, as one student thought, anything to do with the needle becoming a kind of antenna or a honing beacon of spiritual energy. To use my methods, it does not really matter whether the practitioner believes in meridians, *nadis, chi, yin,* or *yang* for him or her to perform this specialized form of acupuncture. You may use these points without having any pre-conceived ideas as to how acupuncture actually works.

Because of my traditional acupuncture training (as well as the use of Western approaches), the rationale for the use of chakra acupuncture (I have not yet been so bold as to call it "chakrapuncture") is based on my traditional belief system. Virtually every acupuncturist would believe in the validity of acupoints as points that have different electrical potential and magnetic properties than areas that surround them. Not every practitioner, however, would believe in the traditional concept of meridians as the invisible channels that transport vital force around the body.

For the purposes of this book, the existence of meridians is taken for granted, simply because the whole concept is easier to explain with this basic belief. My personal concept of meridians has changed over the years—I now believe that they represent holographic extensions of the central and autonomic nervous system. In practical acupuncture terms, it is still possible to utilize the traditional meridian system while not actually believing in its existence. Thousands of acupuncturists do this every day. As I have stated before, until someone can prove beyond any reasonable doubt how *non*-pain relief acupuncture works scientifically, TCM philosophy will still be followed by me and thousands of other practitioners around the world. Please remember that science does not have an answer for everything.

CHAPTER ONE

THE CHAKRAS

You will find a full and detailed description of the subtle bodies (aura) and chakras in my previous book *Healing with the Chakra Energy System,* so a full discussion of the subtle bodies and chakras will not be repeated here. For those of you who have not read *Healing with the Chakra Energy System,* this chapter covers the salient points of the subtle bodies and chakras for you. I have also added some information not found in the first book that pertains specifically to acupuncturists.

THE AURA

There are said to be seven bodies including the Physical Body that make up our aura. They are the Physical, Etheric, Emotional or Astral, Mental, Intuitional, Monadic, and Divine or Spiritual. Different philosophies, individuals, and cultures have given these bodies other names depending on whether they are being discussed in Eastern religious, Hindu, Buddhist, Western spiritual, or New Age terms. There are subdivisions of the Etheric Body, which are extremely important to know—Physical-Etheric and Etheric-Emotional. Some very gifted people have the capability of seeing and interpreting auras (clairvoyants), some people can feel them but not see them, and others just see colors. The acceptance and knowledge of the auras are fundamental precepts in being able to learn about and use the chakras with acupuncture. One cannot exist without the other.

PHYSICAL BODY

Looking at a person from a purely esoteric viewpoint, the physical or dense body has little significance. A yogi or sage, for example, would not be interested in a Physical Body condition—just a person's emotional and spiritual make-up. To the rest of us, it is the body that is treated using physical therapy, manipulation, acupuncture, and massage therapy. Most importantly, the body shows us the signs and symptoms of energy imbalance when tested. In Traditional Chinese Medicine (TCM), a practitioner discovers bodily imbalance through tests such as pulse diagnosis, *hara*-abdominal diagnosis, *tsing* point diagnosis, iris diagnosis, or Listening Post analysis. Symptoms are golden pearls of information that are used to identify the cause of the disease *(dis-ease)*, and they show us how steps can be taken to treat the patient. It is my opinion that most of our ills are caused by imbalance in our Emotional Bodies, and the symptoms of disease are merely housed in the Physical Body. If the chakra points are used, acupuncture affects the subtle bodies, thus treating the etiology of the condition, making acupuncture an equally viable treatment to other traditional Western medical treatments.

ETHERIC BODY

The word *etheric* comes from "ether," meaning the state between energy and matter. This first "invisible" body can be seen by clairvoyants and by most children up to the age of seven, who treat is as a normal part of their vision. The Etheric Body is invisible to most adults, although with diligence it is possible to tune-in to be able to see it. There are two parts to the body: the Physical-Etheric and the Etheric-Emotional. The outer limits of these are approximately one inch and four inches (two and a half and ten centimeters) respectively from the Physical Body. The Etheric Body consists of a network of fine tubular threadlike channels known as the *nadis,* which seem to be related to the cerebro-spinal fluid, endocrine glands, and the autonomic nervous system. This will be fully discussed in the next chapter. The Etheric Body has three main functions that are closely related. It acts as a receiver, assimilator, and transmitter of vital force via the chakras. In other words, it represents a vast clearing house of energy from within outwards and from outwards within.

There is much scientific evidence concerning the existence of the Etheric Body. In 1939, the Soviet scientists Semyon and Valentina Kirlian managed to photograph the aura by using electrical plates that emitted a current. When a person placed his or her hand on the condenser plate, an electrical charge was transferred from the plate to the fingertip, and a photograph was taken. Kirlian photography is still used today, although it has been superseded by aura-imaging techniques developed by Guy Coggins in 1980. The Coggin method uses a special camera to produce a full spectrum of the colors of the aura. Aura-imaging has become hugely popular over the past twenty years. In order to adequately describe a person's health with regard to their auras, a large number of camera shots need to be taken within a short space of time.

EMOTIONAL (ASTRAL) BODY

The third body is called either the Astral Body or Emotional Body because of its involvement with emotions. The outer border of the Emotional (Astral) Body follows roughly the outline shape of the Etheric Body with an outer boundary of approximately ten to twelve inches (twenty-five to thirty centimeters). Barbara Ann Brennan in her excellent book *Hands of Light* writes, "This body interpenetrates the denser bodies that it surrounds. Its colors vary from brilliant clear hues to dark muddy ones. Clear and highly energized feelings such as love, excitement, joy or anger are bright and clear; those feelings that are confused are dark and muddy" (1987). Brennan is a gifted healer and clairvoyant and is able to describe the Emotional (Astral) Body in great detail. The ability to read the Emotional (Astral) Body in this way may take many years of learning experience.

In the Emotional Body, multitudes of different changes are constantly taking place, though an individual may or may not be aware of those changes. Each person is literally bombarded by stimuli from both external and internal sources. The main function of the Emotional Body is to act like a filtration system in a similar way to the Etheric Body. Only when there is imbalance in the Emotional Body—or with the chakras that penetrate it—do we become conscious of a shift from our normal state of being. Changes in the Emotional Body can ultimately lead to changes and hence symptoms in the Physical Body.

MENTAL BODY

The Mental Body may extend as much as thirty inches (seventy-five centimeters) from the Physical Body and is much less dense than the other aural bodies. The substance that composes the Mental Body deals with thoughts and mental processes. They are sometimes called "thought forms." The Mental Body is the region where our thought forms are initiated.

Thus, what we *think* can affect both us and those with whom we are in contact. On one hand, if we lead our lives in a positive and helpful way and think lots of lovely thoughts toward others and ourselves, then we feel well. On the other hand, if we lead our lives with negativity, hatred, pessimism, grief, sorrow, and depressive tendencies, then those thoughts are eventually reflected in our physical make-up. The hackneyed phrase, "You are what you eat," is to a great extent true, and likewise, *you become what you think.* Not only do we feel better internally when we exhibit positive emotions, but we also, after a prolonged period of experiencing positive vibes, experience a permanent change in body chemistry. The blood's chemistry, hormonal levels, and organic secretions all change. This has led many experts in this field to conclude that *we are totally responsible for our own health.*

I would add a couple exceptions to this mind-body philosophy. First, we can only change the vital force within us that hereditary disposition or congenital factors do not govern. Second, we may be affected by environmental factors, such as pollution, that are beyond our control. We are all governed by our genetic make-up and habitat, and some of us will naturally struggle more than others.

The three remaining subtle bodies are usually called Intuitional, Monadic, and Divine, but may be given other names depending on the school of thought. A description of these subtle bodies falls outside the scope of this book, but full descriptions can be found in *Healing with the Chakra Energy System.*

Figure 1.1 shows the auras and major chakras.

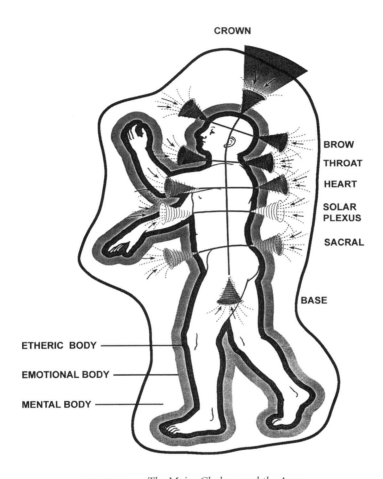

FIGURE 1.1. *The Major Chakras and the Aura*

THE CHAKRAS

The word *chakra* means "wheel" in Sanskrit. The chakras are considered to be *force centers* or whorls of energy permeating from a point on the Physical Body through the layers of the subtle bodies in an ever-increasing, fan-shaped formation. They are rotating vortices of subtle matter and are considered to be the focal points for the reception and transmission of energies. To the clairvoyant, these centers can be seen easily. Each is different in form, make-up, color, and frequency. There are said to be seven major chakras (or force centers), twenty-one minor chakras, and over seven hundred mini-chakras on the body that relate to acupoints and major reflex points.

It is thought that the discovery of chakras stems from Ayurvedic medical philosophy developed over five thousand years ago. If this is true, chakra philosophy is older than Traditional Chinese Medicine (TCM). As with TCM philosophy, the study of the chakras is a lifelong pursuit: no one person can ever hope to have a monopoly on the knowledge and wisdom of the chakras. Over the millennia, different cultures have adopted chakras—each giving the chakras different connotations and importance. The main philosophies involved in chakra knowledge and interpretation are Buddhism, Hindu, Theosophical, Anthropomorphic, and New Age. Due to their esoteric and complex nature, much mysticism surrounds chakras. What I have attempted to do over the past twenty-five years is to make chakras more accessible and easily understood by the practitioner as an untapped source of energy and power to be utilized with many different complementary therapy approaches.

STRUCTURE AND FUNCTIONS

Structure and functions differ from chakra to chakra and also with a person's age. The general shape of a chakra can be likened to an inverted ice cream cone with the pointed end on the Physical Body as an acupoint. The chakra size at the outer border of the Etheric Body is approximately two inches: at the outer border of the Emotional Body it is the size of a saucer; and at the outer border of the Mental Body it is the size of a dinner plate. A full description of the structure of a chakra is available in my first book which was dedicated to hands-on practitioners, who are required to have a very precise awareness of the shapes and forms of chakras for their healing practices. For the general practitioner or acupuncturist, the basics provided here are more than sufficient.

There are three functions of the chakras:

- To vitalize and harmonize the Physical, Etheric, and Emotional Bodies
- To bring about the development of self-consciousness
- To transmit spiritual energy in order to bring the individual into a state of spiritual being

The first function is utilized by the two therapies, acupuncture and biomagnetics, taught in this book. The second function also helps the patient to become more whole in mind, body, and spirit with therapy. The third function remains the prerogative of the meditative arts and the various forms of yoga. According to David Tansley in his book *Radionics and the Subtle Anatomy of Man* (1998), there are three states of chakra imbalance, which often do not appear in the singular but may be a combination of two out of the three . A chakra may be congested, over-stimulated, or simply incoordinated.

1. CONGESTION

Congestion occurs when there is a lack of free flow of energy in the body. Congestion often happens when the vital energy force or *chi* in the area becomes stagnant or sluggish, which in turn may affect blood flow, lymphatic drainage, nerve stimulation, and cerebro-spinal fluid flow. The direction of the congestion can either occur from the outside in or from the inside out. An example of outside in directed congestion would be eating too much saturated fat, causing congestion in the stomach, small bowel, and skin, leading to lymphatic congestion and endocrine imbalance, and finally congestion in the Solar Plexus and Throat chakras. Invading microorganisms can give rise to congestion of the Throat chakra, causing lymphatic congestion in the tonsil and possibly the remainder of the immune system. Although an acupuncturist will not need to feel the

Etheric and Emotional aspects of the chakra, there is a definite difference of feel with a congested chakra compared to the other two states.

2. OVER-STIMULATION

Over-stimulation occurs when too much energy is drawn into and through a particular chakra or chakras. Fevers are an expression of an overactive focal point of energy that is trying to disperse and flow outwards into physical expression. An over-abundant sex drive causes over-stimulation of the Base and Sacral chakras. A person working constantly under fluorescent lighting will have an over stimulated Brow chakra which can cause headaches and a feeling of mental haze.

3. INCOORDINATION

Incoordination occurs between two associated chakras, creating a weakness in one of them and leading to symptoms and poor health. If the Physical and Etheric counterparts of the chakra are not well integrated, debilitation and devitalization will ensue. An example could be edema from a "sluggish" Sacral chakra that has been caused by on overactive Throat chakra (its couple).

THE SEVEN MAJOR CHAKRAS

There has been much debate about where the physical aspects of the major chakras lie and indeed whether or not they are to be found on the anterior or posterior aspect of the body. My experience is that the Crown chakra aspects on the top of the head, the Base chakra aspects at the perineum, and the middle five circle the body around the level of the upper part of the eyes, the throat, the middle of the sternum, the solar plexus, and just below the navel. These horizontal areas exist at the levels of the various diaphragms of the body, namely the sphenoid, the thoracic inlet, the thoracic outlet, the diaphragm, and the pelvic diaphragm.

There seems to be a stronger influence of the girdle of energy situated on both the ventral and dorsal aspects that are situated on the Conception

(Ren Mai) and Governor (Du Mai) meridians. You might call these *points of influence*. Of these two points, the spinal aspect deals mostly with musculo-skeletal, and *yang* imbalance, whereas the ventral aspect deals mostly with organic, emotional, and *yin* imbalance. It is clear, therefore, that when using acupuncture with the chakras, the ventral and spinal aspects are the ones that are most commonly used. If the ventral and spinal points are either forbidden to needle or unavailable for some reason, another point on the same horizontal girdle may be used.

With their relative spinal positions and ventral acupoints, the chakras are as follows:

Chakra	Spinal Level	Spinal Acupoint	Ventral Acupoint
Crown	—	Gov 20	Gov 20
Brow	Occipito-Atlas	Gov 16	Extra 1 (Yintang)
Throat	C7-T1	Gov 14	Con 22
Heart	T6-T7	Gov 10	Con 17
Solar Plexus	T12-L1	Gov 6	Con 14
Sacral	L4-L5	Gov 3	Con 6
Base	Sacro-Coccyx	Gov 2	Con 2

As with my other books, the abbreviations for the Governor and Conception vessels are given as Gov and Con respectively to save confusion that sometimes occurs with the use of GV and CV. Modern acupuncture meridian abbreviation nomenclature is used in this book for all the other meridians. The other anomaly is the positioning of the Base chakra. Strictly speaking there is only one Base chakra point situated at the perineum. Due to obvious anatomical reasons, it is not possible to use this single point in acupuncture (and acupressure), so the points of Gov 2 or Con 2 are used instead. Remember that each chakra horizontally "girdles" the body and the Base chakra "girdles" around the whole of the pubic and genital region so these two very powerful points are representative of the Base chakra for the acupuncturist to use.

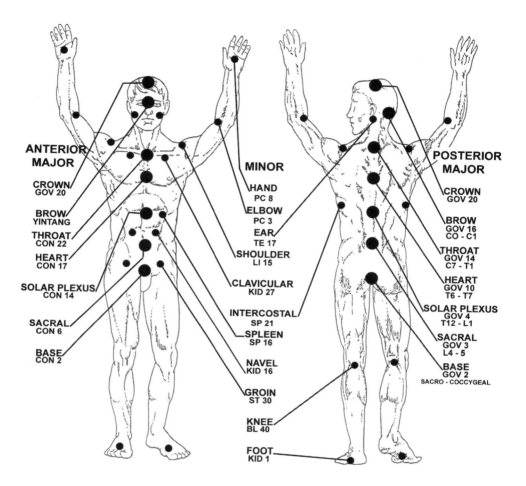

ANTERIOR MAJOR

CROWN
GOV 20

BROW
YINTANG

THROAT
CON 22

HEART
CON 17

SOLAR PLEXUS
CON 14

SACRAL
CON 6

BASE
CON 2

MINOR

HAND
PC 8

ELBOW
PC 3

EAR
TE 17

SHOULDER
LI 15

CLAVICULAR
KID 27

INTERCOSTAL
SP 21

SPLEEN
SP 16

NAVEL
KID 16

GROIN
ST 30

KNEE
BL 40

FOOT
KID 1

POSTERIOR MAJOR

CROWN
GOV 20

BROW
GOV 16
CO - C1

THROAT
GOV 14
C7 - T1

HEART
GOV 10
T6 - T7

SOLAR PLEXUS
GOV 4
T12 - L1

SACRAL
GOV 3
L4 - 5

BASE
GOV 2
SACRO - COCCYGEAL

FIGURE 1.2. *Anatomical Positions of the Major and Minor Chakras*

ASSOCIATIONS AND CORRESPONDENCES OF THE MAJOR CHAKRAS

Each of the seven major chakras is associated with up to twenty-two different correspondences. It is not important to know them all, but a complete study is a fascinating one. Each chakra has a ventral anatomical position, dorsal anatomical position, acupoints—dorsal and ventral, Sanskrit terminology and interpretation, symbol, coupled major chakra, coupled minor chakra, endocrine gland association, organic association, spinal level association, Key points, associated meridians, associated spiritual phenomena, muscular association, autonomic nerve association, color and sound correspondences, and differing number of rotating vortices. Other correspondences that are outside the scope of this book include Element, Life Lesson, Gemstone, Essential Oil, Crystal, Herb, Earth Energy, Planet, and Metal. The Sanskrit terminology presented here is important information for the acupuncturist.

Sanskrit

The Sanskrit language from ancient Indochina is still used today in parts of Mongolia and Tibet. Each major chakra is given Sanskrit terminology. The interpretations are:

- **Crown**—*Sahasrara*—means "thousand-petalled," also "dwelling place without support."
- **Brow**—*Ajna*—means "authority, command and unlimited power."
- **Throat**—*Vishuddha*—means "pure."
- **Heart**—*Anahata*—means "unstricken."
- **Solar Plexus**—*Manipura*—means "the city of gems."
- **Sacral**—*Svadhisthana*—means "dwelling place of the self."
- **Base**—*Muladhara*—means "fountain."

Coupled Major Chakras

In acupuncture, chakra couples are used to balance energy between a chakra and its couple.

- The **Crown** chakra is coupled with the **Base** chakra.
- The **Brow** chakra is *also* coupled with the **Base** chakra.
- The **Throat** chakra is coupled with the **Sacral** chakra.
- The **Heart** chakra is coupled with the **Solar Plexus** chakra.

Please remember that the Base chakra is coupled with both the Crown and the Brow chakras.

COUPLED MINOR CHAKRA

Each major chakra is coupled with one or more of the minor chakras, thus making useful acupuncture combinations.

- The **Crown** chakra is coupled with the **Foot and Hand** chakras.
- The **Brow** chakra is coupled with the **Clavicular and Groin** chakras.
- The **Throat** chakra is coupled with the **Shoulder and Navel** chakras.
- The **Heart** chakra is coupled with the **Ear and Intercostal** chakras.
- The **Solar Plexus** chakra is coupled with the **Spleen** chakra.
- The **Sacral** chakra is *also* coupled with the **Spleen** chakra.
- The **Base** chakra is coupled with the **Knee and Elbow** chakras. (see Figure 1.2)

ENDOCRINE GLAND

Each of the seven major chakras is related to an endocrine gland. Apart from the autonomic nerve system, the endocrine relationship is the most important clinical relationship. The endocrine glands—themselves part of the physical body—have nerve, blood, lymphatic, and energy links to the rest of the body, but also produce hormones that can affect the Physical, Etheric, and Emotional Bodies in an extremely powerful way (see Figure 1.3).

- The **Crown** chakra is linked with the pineal gland.
- The **Brow** chakra is linked with the pituitary, thalamus, and hypothalamus glands.
- The **Throat** chakra is linked with the thyroid and parathyroid glands.
- The **Heart** chakra is linked with the thymus gland.

- The **Solar Plexus** chakra is linked with the pancreas.
- The **Sacral** chakra is linked with the ovaries and testes.
- The **Base** chakra is linked with the adrenal medulla and adrenal cortex.

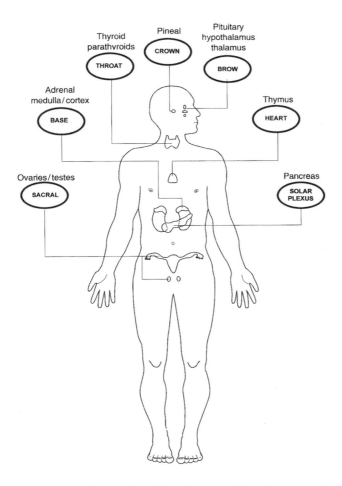

FIGURE 1.3. *Associations of the Major Chakras with the Endocrine Glands*

ASSOCIATED ORGANS

Each major chakra is related to one or more internal organs or parts of the body. This knowledge is vital in clinical terms: once the organic imbalance is known, then the correct chakra may be chosen for treatment. Organ-chakra relationships lie along body's meridian system: an organ and its associated chakra are connected by the main twelve bilateral or by the eight extraordinary meridians.

- The **Crown** chakra is associated with the upper brain (higher functions) and right eye.
- The **Brow** chakra is associated with the lower brain, central nervous system, ears, nose, and left eye.
- The **Throat** chakra is associated with the lungs, bronchus, throat, larynx, pharynx, the upper lymphatic system, and large intestine.
- The **Heart** chakra is associated with the heart, blood circulation, the middle lymphatic system, and the vagus nerve.
- The **Solar Plexus** chakra is associated with the liver, stomach, spleen, pancreas, gall bladder, and the duodenal and jejunum parts of the small intestine.
- The **Sacral** chakra is associated with the reproductive system, lower lymphatic system, and ileum part of the small intestine.
- The **Base** chakra is associated with the spinal column as a whole, kidneys, and bladder.

ASSOCIATED MERIDIANS

Each major chakra is related to one, two, or three meridians. Each minor chakra is related to just one meridian. The knowledge of associated meridians is useful in several ways. Associated meridians may be used as a backup system in energy balancing and treatment. At the commencement of a treatment, a practitioner can needle a source point or stroke the length of a meridian with the flow of energy. At the end of a treatment session, meridians can help balance energy flow in conjunction with general energy balancing. Please note that the meridian relationships as described here are interpreted in relation to my practical years of experience using them.

The meridians that comprise the eight extraordinary ones are included in brackets. These meridians are used in complex, chronic conditions.

- The **Crown** chakra is associated with the Triple Energizer meridian.
- The **Brow** chakra is associated with the Gall Bladder meridian *(Yangwei Mai)*.
- The **Throat** chakra is associated with the Large Intestine and Lung meridians *(Yangchiao Mai)*.
- The **Heart** chakra is associated with the Small Intestine and Heart meridians *(Yin Wei Mai)*.
- The **Solar Plexus** chakra is associated with the Liver and Stomach meridians *(Dai Mai)*.
- The **Sacral** chakra is associated with the Spleen and Pericardium meridians *(Yinchiao Mai)*.
- The **Base** chakra is associated with the Bladder and Kidney meridians *(Conception, Governor* and *Chong Mai)*.

KEY POINTS

The Key points represent those points in acupuncture and the chakra energy system that are needled first in order to "open up" the energy center. Each major chakra has two Key points. Each minor chakra has one Key point. The Key points of chakras are used in a similar way to the Key points of the eight extraordinary meridians. Chakra Key points lie on both the mid-line and the periphery. The discovery of the Key points is based totally on my own research. When doing my acupuncture doctoral thesis in 1986, these points were promulgated as only being of use in acupuncture, but I have since discovered that they are also immensely useful in acupressure. Chakra Key points must be learned: they will be your friends for life!

- **Crown** chakra Key points are TE 5 and Con 4.
- **Brow** chakra Key points are SP 6 and Gov 4.
- **Throat** chakra Key points are LR 5 and Con 6.
- **Heart** chakra Key points are HT 1 and Gov 7.

- **Solar Plexus** chakra Key points are TE 4 and Con 17.
- **Sacral** chakra Key points are PC 3 and Gov 12.
- **Base** chakra Key points are LR 8 and Con 22.

See the illustrations to view the individual chakras.

ASSOCIATED EMOTIONS

Each of the different emotions may be used as diagnostic tools that help identify which chakra is in a state of imbalance. When giving chakra acupuncture, an emotional release is sometimes achieved either during the treatment session or the next day. With deep-seated, emotionally based etiology, the patient must be told to possibly expect such reactions.

- The **Crown** chakra is related to melancholy and several phobias.
- The **Brow** chakra is related to anger and rage.
- The **Throat** chakra is related to shyness, introverted behavior, and paranoia.
- The **Heart** chakra is related to tearfulness, anxiety, depression, and detachedness.
- The **Solar Plexus** chakra is related to depression and anxiety.
- The **Sacral** chakra is related to envy, jealousy, and lust.
- The **Base** chakra is related to insecurity, doubt, and many phobias.

SPIRITUAL

Each of the major chakras is associated with a "spiritual" connotation. Spiritual associations are purely objective and, depending on the reference, different interpretations may be given. Spiritual relationships to each chakra are the original links with the energy centers. For centuries energy centers were used solely in meditation and yoga practices. In short, these are the spiritual aspects related to each chakra:

- The **Crown** chakra is coupled with super-consciousness and "all that is."
- The **Brow** chakra is coupled with intuition.
- The **Throat** chakra is coupled with expression.
- The **Heart** chakra is coupled with love.
- The **Solar Plexus** chakra is coupled with stabilizing, control and "earth."
- The **Sacral** chakra is coupled with pleasure and enjoyment.
- The **Base** chakra is coupled with materialism and "the physical earth plane."

Autonomic Nerve Plexus (ANS)

The relationship between the Autonomic Nerve Plexus (ANS) and the chakras is of huge significance in practical acupuncture. Most health practitioners recognize the autonomic nervous system as having a role in general healing. Further, I have discovered a link between chakra acupuncture and the individual nerve plexus. We already know that there is a strong link between the ANS and endocrine glands—this connection helps us to understand how complex, chronic conditions may be treated using this system. Full details of how to use ANS and endocrine glands in acupunctural treatment are in Chapter Four (see Figure 1.4).

- The **Crown** chakra is not linked with the ANS.
- The **Brow** chakra is linked with the Superior Cervical Ganglion.
- The **Throat** chakra is linked with the Inferior Cervical Ganglion.
- The **Heart** chakra is linked with the Celiac Plexus and Ganglion.
- The **Solar Plexus** chakra is also linked with the Celiac Plexus and Ganglion.
- The **Sacral** chakra is linked with the Inferior Mesenteric Ganglion.
- The **Base** chakra is linked with the Pelvic Plexus.

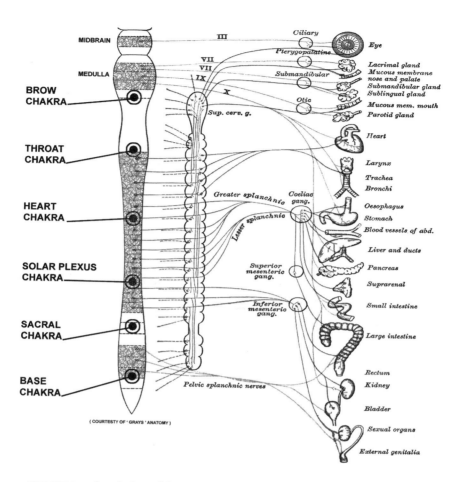

FIGURE 1.4. *Associations of the Major Chakras with the Autonomic Nervous System*

All the above and some of the many other correspondences can be seen in the tables of major and minor chakras: see Tables 1.1 and 1.2. We shall now discuss the individual major and minor chakras.

TABLE 1.1. RELATIONSHIPS OF THE MAJOR CHAKRAS

Major Chakra	Couple	Color	Sound	Meridians	Endocrine Gland	Spinal Level	Body	Emotion	Acup Points	Key Points
Crown	Base	Violet	B	Triple Energizer	Pineal	Cranium	Upper Brain (R) Eye	Melancholy	Gov20	Con 4
Brow	Base	Indigo	A	Gall Bladder	Pituitary	Occipito- Atlas	Lower Brain Nervous System Ears Nose (L) Eye	Anger Rage	Gov16 Extra1	Gov4 SP6
Throat	Sacral	Blue	G	Large Intestine Lung	Thyroid	C7-T1	Bronchial Lungs Vocal Throat Large Bowel	Shyness Paranoia	Gov14 Con22	Con6 LR 5
Heart	Solar Plexus	Green	F	Heart Small Intestine	Thymus	T6-T7	Heart Blood Vagus n.	Tearful Anxiety	Gov10 Con17	Gov7 HT 1
Solar Plexus	Heart	Yellow	E	Liver Stomach	Pancreas	T12-L1	Stomach Liver Spleen	Depression Anxiety	Gov 6 Con14	Con17 TE 4
Sacral	Throat	Orange	D	Spleen Pericardium	Gonads	L4-L5	Repro- ductive System	Jealousy	Gov 3 Con 6	Gov12 PC 3
Base	Crown/ Brow	Red	C	Bladder Kidney	Adrenals	Sacro- Coccyx	Spinal Column Kidneys Bladder	Deep Phobias	Gov 2 Con 2	Con22 LR 8

Major Chakra 1—Crown—Sahasrara

POSITION

There is only one position for the Crown chakra, at acupoint GOV 20, which is situated on the top of the skull in the very center between the eyebrows and the base of the skull and midway between an imaginary line between the front of each ear (see Figure 1.5).

FUNCTION

The Crown chakra is not fully functional until a high degree of inner maturity has been reached. It manifests itself in the pineal gland which medical research shows is more active in children up to the age of seven but slows down later in life. The Crown chakra-related pineal gland affects visual perception. It produces a hormone called melatonin which regulates the light-receptive photoreceptors in the eye's retina. Continuous light decreases melatonin production which may cause symptoms of anxiety or stress. Increased production at night is said to be calming. The pineal gland also produces another hormone—serotonin. Melatonin and serotonin work in a continuous circadian cycle to try and attain our well-being. Serotonin is said to have an important influence in our emotional state where high levels improve the mood by inducing calm and lifting depression. Thus, the Crown chakra is used extensively in yoga and the meditative arts. The Crown chakra appears to govern the upper motor neuron region of the brain and the right eye and is the link between a person and his or her spiritual plane of existence through to the Divine body.

The Crown chakra is sometimes called the "thousand-petalled lotus" because of the shape of its central vortex. There are, in fact, 972 small rotating vortices, not one thousand. Care should be taken when needling this point. Patients may feel disoriented or woozy, and there is a possibility of becoming detached from reality. Side effects, however, are a rare occurrence if the patient is lying down and the needle is only *in situ* for a maximum of fifteen minutes.

The associated meridian is the Triple Energizer. The related major chakra is the Base chakra. Related minor chakras are the Foot and Hand chakras. The Key points are TE 5 and Con 4.

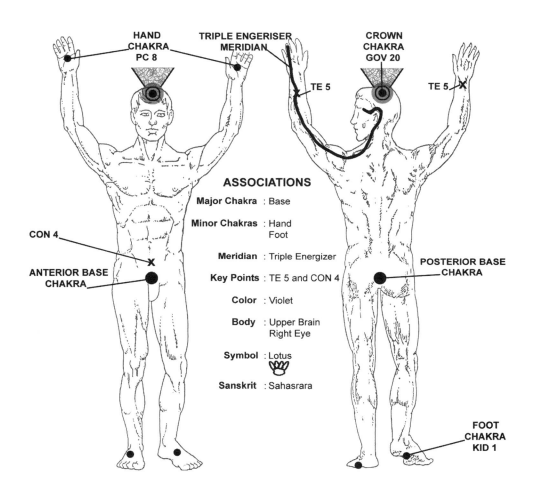

ASSOCIATIONS

Major Chakra : Base

Minor Chakras : Hand
Foot

Meridian : Triple Energizer

Key Points : TE 5 and CON 4

Color : Violet

Body : Upper Brain
Right Eye

Symbol : Lotus

Sanskrit : Sahasrara

SUPERCONSCIOUS : ALL THAT IS

FIGURE 1.5. *Associations of the Crown Chakra*

SYMPTOMATOLOGY

Symptoms of Crown chakra disorder include vertigo, tinnitus, hypertension, migraine (mostly right-sided), headache, symptoms of upper motor neuron diseases, e.g., multiple sclerosis (MS), seasonal affected disorder (SAD), and brittle nails.

The list of symptoms that warrant treatment via the Crown chakra is not extensive. Symptoms appear and are treated in correlation with other affected chakras, such as the Brow chakra in the treatment of headaches, eyestrain, dizziness, tinnitus, temporomandibular joint disorder (TMJ), nasal symptoms, and vertigo.

MAJOR CHAKRA 2—BROW—AJNA

POSITION

The Brow chakra is situated at the *inion,* which is the junction of the base of the skull and the atlas (*occipito-atlas* junction). The acupoint there is Gov 16. The frontal position is midway between the eyes at point Extra 1 *(Yintang)*. The Extra 1 point is sometimes called Gov 24.5 (see Figure 1.6).

FUNCTION

In esoteric literature, the Brow chakra is said to represent the third or hidden eye. The term third eye is appropriate, as the Brow chakra is most useful in treating conditions of perception—both physical and emotional. Extra-sensory perception and clairvoyance externalize through the third eye chakra which is therefore important in intuition. The Brow deals with the personality of the person, and it externalizes as the pituitary gland which is the "master gland" of the endocrine system. Many texts incorrectly associate the Brow center to the pineal gland and the Crown to the pituitary. The Brow chakra is associated with mental vision and intuitiveness, not literal vision—*insight* not *sight.*

Using acupuncture to influence the Brow center affects hormonal secretions which is impossible to do using the Crown chakra. Particularly useful in the treatment of hormonal imbalance, the Brow chakra governs the lower brain, central nervous system, left eye, nose, and ears. The anterior chakra at acupoint Extra 1 *(Yintang)* is the equivalent to the first point on the bladder meridian (BL1) and shares many of its functions. The relationship between Extra 1 and BL1 is explained further in Chapter Four.

The Key points are SP 6 and Gov 4 and the Gall Bladder is the associated meridian.

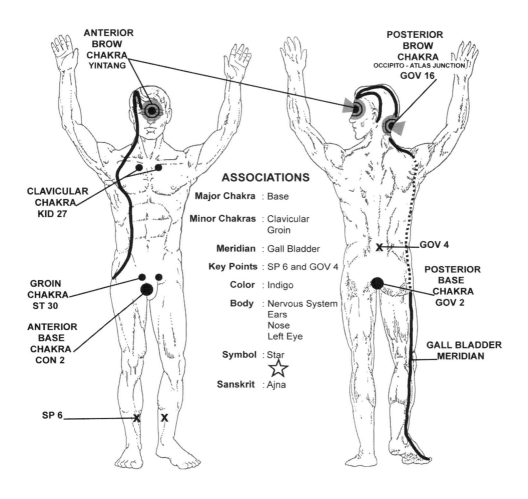

ANTERIOR
BROW
CHAKRA
YINTANG

POSTERIOR
BROW
CHAKRA
OCCIPITO - ATLAS JUNCTION
GOV 16

CLAVICULAR
CHAKRA
KID 27

ASSOCIATIONS

Major Chakra : Base

Minor Chakras : Clavicular
Groin

GOV 4

Meridian : Gall Bladder

Key Points : SP 6 and GOV 4

POSTERIOR
BASE
CHAKRA
GOV 2

GROIN
CHAKRA
ST 30

Color : Indigo

Body : Nervous System
Ears
Nose
Left Eye

ANTERIOR
BASE
CHAKRA
CON 2

GALL BLADDER
MERIDIAN

Symbol : Star
☆

Sanskrit : Ajna

SP 6

INTUITION : INTELLECTUAL

FIGURE 1.6. *Associations of the Brow Chakra*

SYMPTOMATOLOGY

Symptoms of the Brow chakra include migraine, chronic and acute catarrh, sinusitis, altered hearing, deafness, arthritis of the upper cervical spine, temporomandibular joint disorder (TMJ), Ménière's disease, vertigo, dizziness, light-headedness, headaches, stress-related symptoms, anxiety-related symptoms, and symptoms of some motor neuron diseases, e.g.,

Parkinson's, rage, anger, and shyness. As with all the dual-based chakras, the dorsal chakra helps the most in the treatment of musculo-skeletal conditions. The anterior chakra helps the most in treatment of organic and neurological conditions. Needling both aspects of the chakra at Extra 1 and Gov 16 is probably the most powerful anti-stress and relaxation duo of points in the whole body.

Major Chakra 3—Throat—Vishuddha

POSITION

The Throat or *Vishuddha* chakra is situated at the junction of the seventh cervical and first thoracic vertebra (C7-T1) at acupoint Gov 14. The anterior aspect is at point Con 22 in the center of the sternal notch (see Figure 1.7).

FUNCTION

The Throat chakra is a powerful chakra and one of the most actively used in acupuncture, next to the Base chakra. The Throat chakra is thought to be the lowest chakra of the higher self and manifests physically in the thyroid and parathyroid glands. The Throat chakra is often congested when organisms and viruses invade, producing symptoms including sore throat and tonsillitis. The Throat chakra tends to be the body's first line of defense. The long-term affect of the suppression of the thyroid and parathyroid glands by drug therapy may be a contributing factor in multifactorial symptomatic conditions such as glandular fever, chronic fatigue syndrome or myalgic encephalomyelitis (ME), and chronic asthma: treating the Throat chakra can help these conditions. When the Throat chakra is in a state of imbalance, people cannot express themselves easily and may act shy, reclusive, and introverted. Imbalance to the Throat chakra may be caused by a sudden emotional shock such as grief.

Associated with the large bowel and lungs, the Throat chakra is involved with *excretion* at all levels. The Throat chakra also governs the excretion of waste thoughts and "hang-ups" (not phobias). Associations with the minor chakras of the Shoulder and Navel heighten the Throat chakra's influence on waste excretion.

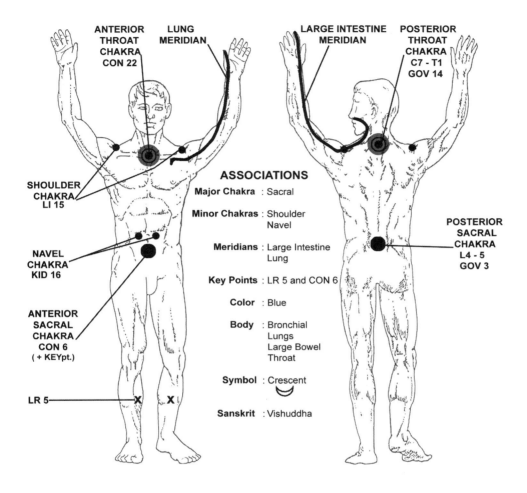

ASSOCIATIONS

Major Chakra : Sacral

Minor Chakras : Shoulder
Navel

Meridians : Large Intestine
Lung

Key Points : LR 5 and CON 6

Color : Blue

Body : Bronchial
Lungs
Large Bowel
Throat

Symbol : Crescent

Sanskrit : Vishuddha

EXPRESSION : EXCRETION

FIGURE 1.7. *Associations of the Throat Chakra*

Key points of the Throat chakra are LR 5—found two cun superior to SP 6 on the medial aspect of the tibia and Con 6—one and one-half cun inferior to the umbilicus. A cun is sometimes called a "Chinese inch" and is equivalent to the width of the thumb. The associated meridians are the Large Intestine and Lung.

SYMPTOMATOLOGY

Symptoms of the Throat Chakra include migraine, acute and chronic sore throat, tonsillitis, asthma, loss of taste, acute and chronic bronchitis and other respiratory tract infections, laryngitis, colitis, irritable bowel syndrome (IBS), ileocecal valve syndrome, shyness, introverted behavior, paranoia, and chronic skin lesions such as eczema.

The posterior aspect of this chakra, situated at the C/T junction, is very useful in the treatment of stress that creates neck muscle tension, fibrosis, and some patients with frozen shoulder or *adhesive capsulitis.*

MAJOR CHAKRA 4—HEART—ANAHATA

POSITION

The Heart or *Anahata* chakra is situated at the center of the thoracic spine at level T6-T7 (Gov 10). The anterior aspect is situated half way down the sternum at Con 17 (see Figure 1.8).

FUNCTION

In contrast to the Throat chakra, the Heart chakra is one of the least used in clinical acupuncture concerning physical conditions. The great significance of the Heart chakra is in the treatment of emotional states. Although the associated endocrine gland is the thymus, there seems to be little use for this relationship in clinical acupuncture. When this chakra is overactive, it can produce an amoral, irresponsible individual. Energy flooding uncontrolled into this chakra can have a devastating affect on someone's personality, especially with affairs of the heart! Over-stimulation can produce the idyllic state of sheer bliss of falling in love which may give one an almost "out of this world" type of feeling. People may cry easily and become easily upset. This is the chakra of the "giggler" and of those who weep when telling their sorrowful story at the consultation. Executives and entrepreneurs have great strain put on their Heart chakra and can suffer heart trouble as a consequence. Doctors and therapists in the caring professions who cannot detach themselves from their patients are in a similar plight.

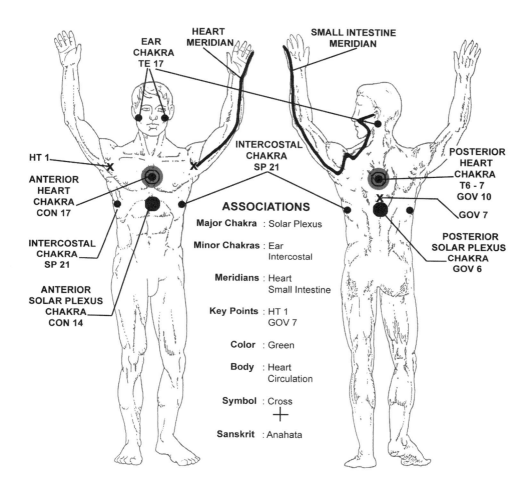

EAR CHAKRA TE 17

HEART MERIDIAN

SMALL INTESTINE MERIDIAN

HT 1

ANTERIOR HEART CHAKRA CON 17

INTERCOSTAL CHAKRA SP 21

INTERCOSTAL CHAKRA SP 21

ANTERIOR SOLAR PLEXUS CHAKRA CON 14

POSTERIOR HEART CHAKRA T6 - 7 GOV 10

GOV 7

POSTERIOR SOLAR PLEXUS CHAKRA GOV 6

ASSOCIATIONS

Major Chakra : Solar Plexus

Minor Chakras : Ear
Intercostal

Meridians : Heart
Small Intestine

Key Points : HT 1
GOV 7

Color : Green

Body : Heart
Circulation

Symbol : Cross

Sanskrit : Anahata

ANXIETY : DETACHMENT : LOVE

FIGURE 1.8. *Associations of the Heart Chakra*

The associated meridians are the Heart and Small Intestine, and the Key points are HT 1 and Gov 7.

SYMPTOMATOLOGY

Symptoms of the Heart chakra include benign tumors and growths, thoracic scoliosis—either idiopathic or congenital, heart conditions ranging from congestive heart failure to simple circulatory imbalance, palpitation, tachycardia, bradycardia, angina, varicosities, tearfulness, anxiety, insularity, and introversion.

MAJOR CHAKRA 5—SOLAR PLEXUS—MANIPURA

POSITION

The Solar Plexus chakra is situated at the junction of the thoracic and lumbar spine at T12-L1 (Gov 6). The ventral aspect is located just below the xiphoid process of the sternum at Con 14 (see Figure 1.9).

FUNCTION

The Solar Plexus chakra represents a vast clearing house of energies found below the diaphragm. In most people the Solar Plexus chakra is either over- stimulated by the sheer pace of life or congested by eating denatured or additive-filled foods. Over-stimulation and congestion can cause nervous disorders and consequent stomach, liver, gall bladder, pancreas, and spleen conditions. If the energy imbalance of the Solar Plexus chakra becomes chronic, a decrease in the energy potential of the body's immune system and conditions such as chronic fatigue syndrome or myalgic encephalomyelitis (ME) ensue. Weakness in the abdominal area due to a congested Solar Plexus chakra can cause slight scoliosis or muscular imbalances resulting in spasm of the erector spinae group of muscles. Such physical misalignment may further affect the cervical and lumbar spine which attempt to compensate for the mid-thoracic region. Therefore, the Solar Plexus is vital to the treatment of many organic and emotional conditions. The associated endocrine gland is the insulin-producing pancreas, which enables sugar metabolism.

The associated meridians are the Liver and Stomach. The Key points are TE 4 and Con 17.

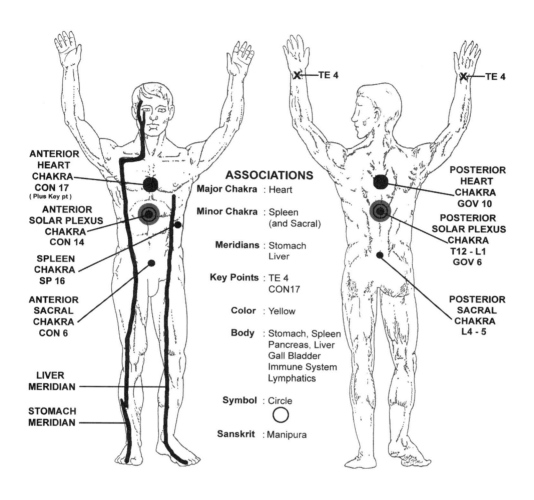

ANTERIOR
HEART
CHAKRA
CON 17
(Plus Key pt)

ANTERIOR
SOLAR PLEXUS
CHAKRA
CON 14

SPLEEN
CHAKRA
SP 16

ANTERIOR
SACRAL
CHAKRA
CON 6

LIVER
MERIDIAN

STOMACH
MERIDIAN

ASSOCIATIONS

Major Chakra : Heart

Minor Chakra : Spleen
(and Sacral)

Meridians : Stomach
Liver

Key Points : TE 4
CON17

Color : Yellow

Body : Stomach, Spleen
Pancreas, Liver
Gall Bladder
Immune System
Lymphatics

Symbol : Circle

Sanskrit : Manipura

TE 4
TE 4

POSTERIOR
HEART
CHAKRA
GOV 10

POSTERIOR
SOLAR PLEXUS
CHAKRA
T12 - L1
GOV 6

POSTERIOR
SACRAL
CHAKRA
L4 - 5

STABILISING : CONTROL : EARTH

FIGURE 1.9. *Associations of the Solar Plexus Chakra*

SYMPTOMATOLOGY

Symptoms of the Solar Plexus chakra include conditions such as eczema
and acne, stomach ulcers, cancerous growths, hepatitis, diabetes, gall bladder colic, indigestion and dyspepsia, infections of the glandular system

as a whole, glandular fever, chronic fatigue syndrome or myalgic encephalomyelitis (ME), allergies, hay fever, small intestine spasms, irritable bowel syndrome (IBS), worry, depression, and anxiety.

Diabetes and cancer are the most common chronic conditions associated with the Solar Plexus chakra. Although there are often physical and chemical causes of these diseases, symptoms are often precipitated by imbalance in the emotional and mental bodies. Diabetes might be caused by a person not allowing enough sweetness and love to enter his or her life. Holding on to emotions of anger, fear, and hatred may be a contributing factor in the etiology of cancer. Conventional medical treatment works well to resolve outward symptoms but does not treat the underlying problems. Importantly, unless you are a registered medical practitioner, you must never attempt to treat diabetes or cancer. However, there is nothing wrong with treating a person who has these conditions as long as the patient is fully aware that treatment is not a cure.

The Solar Plexus is often called the seat of our emotions. The sentiment behind the phrase "having a gut feeling" stems from the energy of the Solar Plexus chakra. "Butterflies" in the abdomen in times of stress may also indicate an overactive Solar Plexus chakra. This nervous sensation usually disappears when relaxation occurs, except in the case of chronic thoracic inflammation which may cause ongoing pain throughout the stomach and diaphragm from such conditions as inflamed thoracic scoliosis, ankylosing spondylitis, or rheumatoid arthritis.

MAJOR CHAKRA 6—SACRAL—SVADHISTHANA

POSITION

The Sacral chakra is situated at the junction of Lumbar 4-5 near the base of the spine (Gov 3). The ventral aspect is Con 6 which is located one and one-half cun (two finger widths) below the umbilicus. This frontal point is also called the *hara*—a point that is widely used in meditative practices, yoga, martial arts, and subtle energy exercise such as *Aikido* and *Tai Chi* (see Figure 1.10).

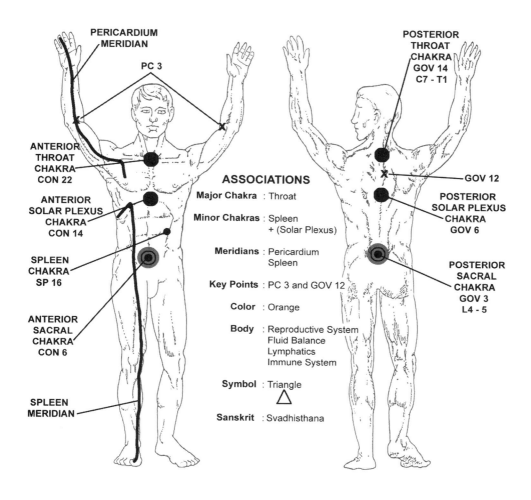

PLEASURE : ENJOYMENT : SEXUAL

FIGURE 1.10. *Associations of the Sacral Chakra*

FUNCTION

This chakra is said to rule the reproductive system and the control of water within the body. In some texts, the Sacral chakra is known as the Spleen or Navel chakra. My research and subsequent experience contradicts this nomenclature, since the Spleen and Navel are both minor chakras with separate functions from the Sacral chakra. The main use of the Sacral chakra is in the treatment of reproductive, gynecological, and obstetric conditions. The Sacral chakra is also associated with the lower third of the small intestine and is therefore involved with the assimilation and absorption of food. Despite being involved with water control, the kidneys do not appear to be associated with the Sacral chakra. The kidneys, in my opinion, are linked with the Base chakra. Nevertheless it cannot be denied that a Sacral chakra imbalance affects water rhythms within the body. The Shamanic teachings from Native Americans associate all water creatures with the Sacral chakra. Bodily circadian and monthly cycles are governed by this chakra, including the menstrual cycle. Other texts link the Sacral chakra with the adrenal glands. Extensive research and clinical practice on my part has shown that the endocrine link with Sacral Chakra is with the uterus and gonads, not the adrenals. If the Sacral chakra is under active and sluggish, then there is an urge to eat excessively, which may result in a lowered sex drive in some people. An ongoing imbalance of the Sacral chakra leads to obesity, food intolerance, chronic skin conditions, and possible impotence. Traditional wisdom tells us to regain sacred or *sacral* equilibrium through dance, laughter (a good belly laugh), yoga, breathing exercises, and visualization of orange light.

The associated meridians are the Spleen and Pericardium, and the Key points are PC 3 and Gov 12.

SYMPTOMATOLOGY

Symptoms of the Sacral chakra include low vitality, some intestinal and gastric conditions, irritable bowel syndrome, chronic tiredness and lethargy, impotence, chronic sore throats, menstrual and menopausal conditions, edema, swollen ankles, some rheumatoid factor conditions, and imbalanced body temperature—including cold feet and chilblains.

MAJOR CHAKRA 7—BASE—MULADHARA

POSITION

Because the exact position of the Base chakra is at the perineum, an extremely delicate part of the body, alternate points are used. Remember,

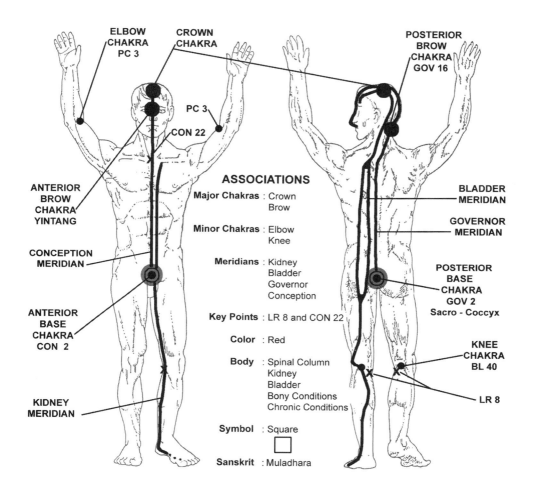

ASSOCIATIONS

Major Chakras : Crown
Brow

Minor Chakras : Elbow
Knee

Meridians : Kidney
Bladder
Governor
Conception

Key Points : LR 8 and CON 22

Color : Red

Body : Spinal Column
Kidney
Bladder
Bony Conditions
Chronic Conditions

Symbol : Square

Sanskrit : Muladhara

MATERIAL : PHYSICAL : GROUNDING : ANCESTRY

FIGURE 1.11. *Associations of the Base Chakra*

an area of influence girdles the body at each chakra level, so for practical purposes the ventral point of Con 2 (upper crest of the symphysis pubis) and posterior point of Gov 2 (sacro-coccygeal junction) are equally useful. Due to the delicate nature of the area, some acupuncturists and patients remain reluctant to use these two points, but the Base chakra is the most important chakra in clinical terms and is used more than any other chakra in everyday acupuncture. Once the importance of the Base chakra acupoints is understood, there are few problems gaining a patient's permission to work in the region near the perineum. However, permission from the patient must *always* be sought prior to needling—it must never be taken for granted (see Figure 1.11).

FUNCTION

The Base chakra (sometimes called the Root chakra) is used more than any other chakra in everyday clinical work because it can be used to treat *anything* that is chronic. In isolation or in combination with other relevant chakras the Base chakra can be used to treat chronic mechanical, osteoarthritis, hereditary, and deep emotional conditions. The Base chakra is responsible for anchoring the body on the physical plane and providing a channel for the will to express itself. In spiritual terms it is relatively dormant and inactive in the general population, but its activity is on the increase due to the stress of modern living. The Base chakra is associated with the adrenal medulla and cortex, the former being responsible for the production of adrenaline and the latter, cortisone. The Base chakra is used in the treatment of deep- seated hereditary and miasmatic weakness and is the focal point for any condition concerning the spinal column and kidneys. Psychosomatic problems—such as the will to live being at a low ebb—are also associated with this chakra.

The associated meridians are the Kidney and Bladder, and the Key points are LR 8 (situated on the medial aspect of the knee) and Con 22 (situated in the sternal notch).

SYMPTOMATOLOGY

Symptoms of the Base chakra include osteoarthritis, ankylosing spondylitis, rheumatoid arthritis, nephritis, chronic cystitis, chronic prostatitis, gravitational ulcers, Scheuermann's disease, other bone diseases, depression, lethargy, chronic tiredness, chronic spinal conditions, and some phobias.

We shall now consider the twenty-one minor chakras.

THE TWENTY-ONE MINOR CHAKRAS

Though many authors discuss the major chakras in their books, most neglect to discuss the minor chakras in depth. Usually only brief mentions based on David Tansley's original illustration of their positioning in *Radionics and the Subtle Anatomy of Man* are made. Unfortunately, most of the positions given in that book are, in my opinion, incorrect. After several years of research I have ascertained the location and function of the twenty-one minor chakras, and I share my findings in both *Healing with the Chakra Energy System* and this book.

Why are these chakras called "minor chakras"? Why are there twenty-one? These chakras are called "minor" because they are inferior in energetic significance to the major chakras yet have a more potent affect and more usefulness than most "ordinary" acupoints. There are twenty-one minor chakras because there are ten bilateral points—plus the odd one—the Spleen chakra.

In discussing the major chakras, it was said that each point on the physical body was a gateway to our higher selves and that each point represented powerful acupoints. Clairvoyants tell us that each of the major chakras has twenty-one concentric circles or whorls of energy. They also tell us that the minor chakras are the second most important set of acupoint, trigger, or reflected points on the body because they are said to have fourteen concentric circles of energy. The important "Great" points such as LI 4, LR 3, and SP 6 are said to have seven concentric circles, and the remainder of the acupoints and reflex points have between two and five depending on their energetic significance. This whole field of energy medicine merits further investigation.

Although the minor centers are powerful points, there is no evidence of astral or spiritual connections except to the Emotional Body limit of the Etheric Body. Minor chakras may therefore be considered as reflex points or "reflected" parts of the seven major chakras. Though there are many characteristics of the minor chakras the main characteristic (discussed in Chapter Three) is the ability to relieve pain.

Positions	Minor Chakra	Acupoint
1	Spleen chakra	SP 16 (L)
2 and 3	Foot chakra	KID 1
4 and 5	Hand chakra	PC 8
6 and 7	Knee chakra	BL 40
8 and 9	Elbow chakra	PC 3
10 and 11	Groin chakra	ST 30
12 and 13	Clavicular chakra	KID 27
14 and 15	Shoulder chakra	LI 15
16 and 17	Navel chakra	KID 16
18 and 19	Ear chakra	TE 17
20 and 21	Intercostal chakra	SP 21

I have assigned each of the minor chakras with my own simple nomenclature. Apart from the Spleen chakra, which is unique in many ways, all are bilateral points and appear mostly on the antero-lateral aspect of the torso and limbs. It should also be noted that each of the acupoints which constitute the physical counterpart of each minor chakra is a "powerful" point in its own right. It is no coincidence that three of the minor chakra points are situated on the kidney meridian, and two are on the pericardium meridian. These vessels represent two of the deepest of the body's energies in ancestry and quality.

As with the seven major chakras, the twenty bilateral minor chakras each have a coupled minor chakra on the same side of the body, e.g., right with right and left with left. For example, the couple of the left Hand chakra is the left Foot chakra. When a chakra is in a state of energy imbalance and is being treated, its couple is also needled to create an energy balance. With each minor chakra, a Key point exists that is used to "open up" the energy flow prior to treatment: the related meridian is also used to enhance the treatment, either by needling the Source point or by stroking it with the flow of energy. There are many other relationships similar to the major chakras: symptomatology—local, general, color, sound, pitch, frequency, vibrational rate, and homeopathic link. Sound pitch, frequency, vibrational rate, and homeopathic remedies fall outside the scope of this book. Below is an abbreviated table for those associations that are vital in the practice of chakra acupuncture.

TABLE 1.2 RELATIONSHIP OF THE MINOR CHAKRAS

Minor Chakra	Coupled Minor Chakra	Coupled Major Chakra	Meridian(s)	Key Point	Color
Spleen	Nil	Solar Plexus, Sacral	Spleen Lung	GOV 8	Yellow
Foot	Hand	Crown	Kidney	HT 6	Violet
Hand	Foot	Crown	Heart	KID 3	Violet
Knee	Elbow	Base	Bladder	SI 7	Red
Elbow	Knee	Base	Small Intestine	BL 59	Red
Groin	Clavicular	Brow	Liver	PC 7	Indigo
Clavicular	Groin	Brow	Pericardium	LR 8	Indigo
Shoulder	Navel	Throat	Large Intestine	ST 40	Blue
Navel	Shoulder	Throat	Stomach	LI 11	Blue
Ear	Intercostal	Heart	Gall Bladder	TE 4	Green
Intercostal	Ear	Heart	Triple Energizer	GB 37	Green

The following are descriptions of the individual minor chakras:

SPLEEN CHAKRA

The Spleen chakra is located at point SP 16 (L) situated four cun lateral to Con 11 which is three cun superior to the umbilicus. The Key point is at Gov 8 situated between T9 and T10. The Spleen chakra is said to be the major amongst the minors and behaves differently than any of the other minor chakras. Closely associated with the Solar Plexus and Sacral chakras, the full benefit of treatment is obtained when all three are used together (see Figure 1.12).

Symptomatology

The Spleen chakra follows both orthodox and TCM lines when it comes to symptoms caused by energy imbalance:

1. Symptoms of an auto-immune system imbalance,
2. Leukocyte imbalance,
3. Infection of any kind,
4. Lymphatic circulation and obstruction,
5. Uterine imbalance.

Therefore, the following named conditions can be caused by a Spleen chakra imbalance and can be treated either in isolation or in combination with the coupled majors of the Solar Plexus and Sacral chakras: Glandular fever, children's skin conditions, chronic tonsillitis, breast tumors, pre-menstrual irregularities, leukorrhea, menopausal symptoms, edema, lethargy, chronic fatigue syndrome or myalgic encephalomyelitis (ME), allergies, and viral infections.

The remaining twenty minor chakras will now be discussed. The main role of a minor chakra is pain relief, but each chakra also has several other local and general uses. Each chakra may be treated as a unit although it is usually treated with its coupled chakra. You should learn the couples by heart, but with practice they will become second nature to you.

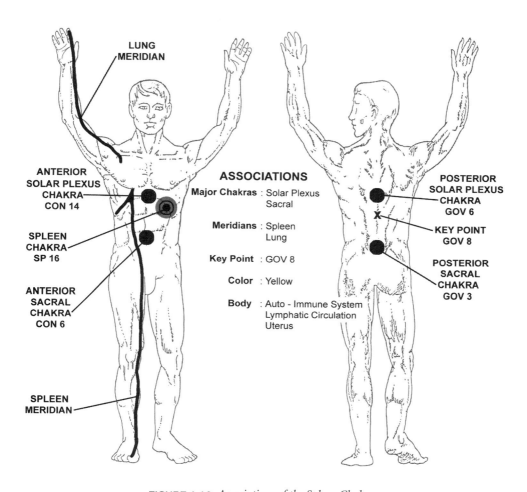

FIGURE 1.12. *Associations of the Spleen Chakra*

FOOT CHAKRA

The Foot chakra is situated at KID 1, the only meridian acupoint on the sole of the foot, in the depression at the junction of the anterior and middle third of the sole between the second and third metatarso-phalangeal joints. As you probably know, this point can be quite painful to needle so insert it quickly and do not get in the way of the patient's kicking leg! It is such a useful and powerful point that this small inconvenience should be tolerated. The Key point is at Ht 6, situated half a cun superior to Shenmen

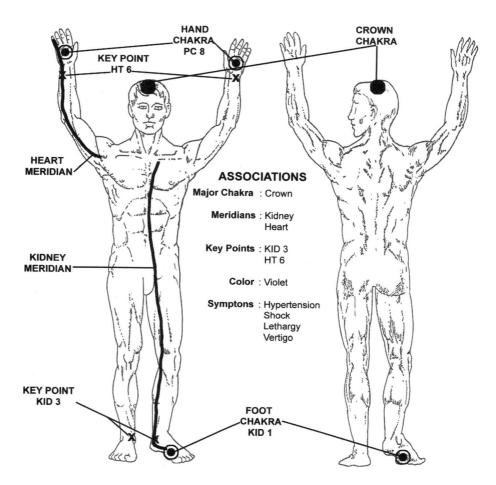

FIGURE 1.13. *Associations of the Hand and Foot Chakras*

(HT 7) which is just superior to the pisiform bone. It is associated with the Kidney meridian and coupled with the Crown and Hand chakras (see Figure 1.13).

Local Symptoms

Local symptoms of the Foot chakra are metatarsalgia, foot pain, dropped arches, callous formation, edema of the foot, and heel spur.

General Symptoms

General symptoms of the Foot chakra are hypertension, infantile convulsions, epilepsy, shock, fainting, lethargy, dizziness, headaches, migraine, and insomnia.

HAND CHAKRA

The Hand chakra is situated in the very center of the palm at PC 8 (often called the stigmata point). The Key point is KID 3, situated midway between the tip of the medial malleolus and the Achilles tendon. This chakra is associated with the Heart meridian and coupled with the Foot and Crown chakras.

Local Symptoms

Local symptoms of the Hand chakra include plantar fasciitis, Dupuytren's contracture, and skin infections local to the hand and nails.

General Symptoms

General symptoms are the same as those of the Foot chakra (Figure 1.13).

KNEE CHAKRA

The Knee chakra is situated in the center of the popliteal fossa at point BL 40. The Key point is SI 7, situated five cun proximal to the wrist on the ulnar border. This chakra is associated with the Bladder meridian and is coupled with the Elbow and Base chakras.

Local Symptoms

Local symptoms of the Knee chakra include sciatica, knee bursitis, knee weakness and discomfort, Osgood Schlatter's syndrome, and osteoarthritis of the knee especially at the lateral border.

General Symptoms

General symptoms of the Knee chakra include cold feet, poor leg circulation, hip pain, sacral and sacroiliac pain and joint changes, lumbar spine pain and joint changes, and cystitis.

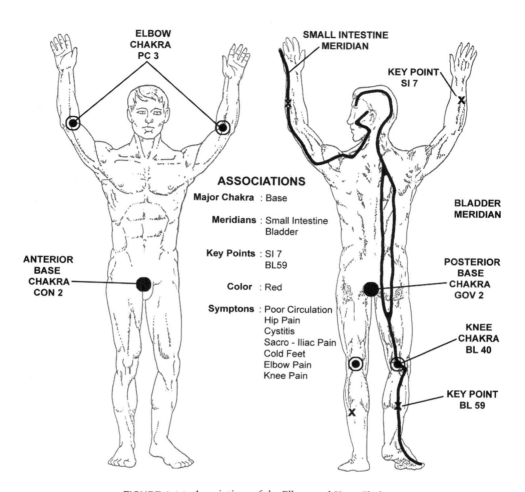

FIGURE 1.14. *Associations of the Elbow and Knee Chakras*

ELBOW CHAKRA

The Elbow chakra is situated at the center of the cubital fossa on the anterior aspect of the elbow joint at point PC 3. The Key point is BL 59, situated three cun superior to BL 60 posterior to the fibula. It is associated with the Small Intestine meridian and is coupled with the Knee and Base chakras.

Local Symptoms

Symptoms of the Elbow chakra include elbow joint pain, elbow joint stiffness, and acute, chronic tennis elbow, also known as epicondylitis.

General Symptoms

General symptoms of the Elbow chakra are the same as those of the Knee chakra with the addition of palpitation and angina (Figure 1.14).

GROIN CHAKRA

The Groin chakra is positioned two cun lateral to Con 2 at the level of the superior aspect of the symphysis pubis at point ST 30. The Key point is at PC 7, situated in the center of the anterior wrist crease. The Groin chakra is associated with the Liver meridian and is coupled with the Clavicular and Brow chakras.

Local Symptoms

Local symptoms of the Groin chakra include hip pain, stiffness, joint changes, loin area circulation imbalance, inguinal hernia, testicular conditions, weak libido, and general urogenital symptoms.

General Symptoms

General symptoms of the Groin chakra include low blood pressure, non-psychosomatic asthma, vomiting, and chest pain.

CLAVICULAR CHAKRA

The Clavicular chakra is situated at the medial end of the clavicle at acupoint KID 27. The Key point is LR 8 (same as the Base chakra) which is situated at the medial aspect of the knee joint. The associated meridian is the Pericardium, and it is coupled with the Groin and Brow chakras.

Local Symptoms

Local symptoms of the Clavicular chakra include chest pain, thyroid imbalance, lower cervical stiffness, sternal pain, and sterno-clavicular joint pain.

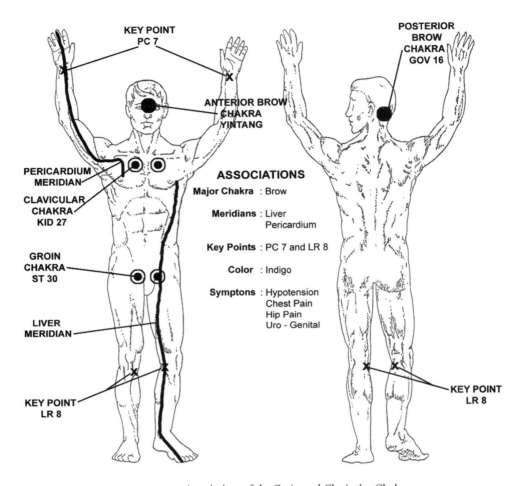

FIGURE 1.15. *Associations of the Groin and Clavicular Chakras*

General Symptoms

General symptoms of the Clavicular chakra are the same as those of the Groin chakra with the addition of generalized bony abnormalities due to imbalance of calcium metabolism, e.g., Scheuermann's disease and ankylosing spondylitis (See Figure 1.15).

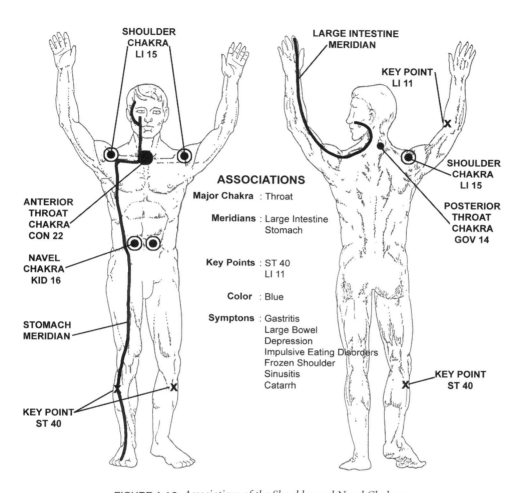

FIGURE 1.16. *Associations of the Shoulder and Navel Chakras*

SHOULDER CHAKRA

The Shoulder chakra is a very powerful chakra situated at the anterior and inferior aspect of the acromion-clavicular joint at acupoint LI 15. The Key point is ST 40 which is situated eight cun inferior to the knee joint just posterior to the fibula. The associated meridian is the Large Intestine, and it is coupled with the Navel and Throat chakras.

Local Symptoms

Local symptoms of the Shoulder chakra are pain in the shoulder joint, with or without joint changes and stiffness, and frozen shoulder.

General Symptoms

General symptoms of the Shoulder chakra include gastritis, small and large bowel pain, constipation, chronic diarrhea, diverticulitis, irritable bowel syndrome, compulsive eating disorders, and depression.

NAVEL CHAKRA

The Navel chakra is situated just lateral to the umbilicus (navel) at point KID 16. The Key point is LI 11 situated at the lateral aspect of the elbow joint. The Naval chakra is associated with the Stomach meridian and is coupled with the Shoulder and Throat chakras.

Local Symptoms

Local symptoms of the Naval chakra include localized pain around the lower abdomen, irritable bowel syndrome, and ileocecal valve syndrome.

General Symptoms

General symptoms of the Naval chakra are those of the Shoulder chakra with the addition of general weariness and some symptoms associated with anorexia (See Figure 1.16).

EAR CHAKRA

The Ear chakra is situated just posterior to the ear lobe at acupoint TE 17. The Key point is TE 4 which is found in the centre of the posterior wrist crease. It is the only chakra whose Key point lies on the same meridian as the chakra. Associated with the Gall Bladder meridian, the Ear chakra is coupled with the Intercostal and Heart chakras.

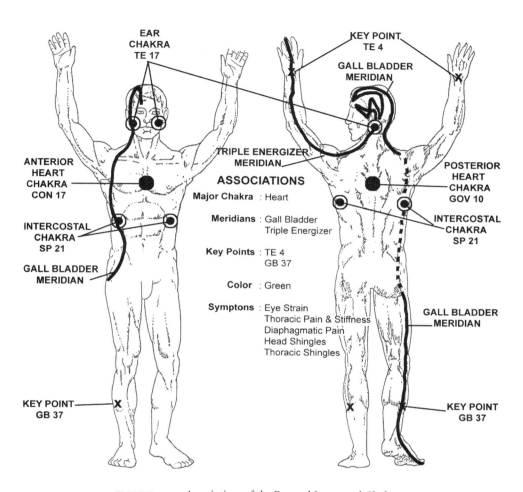

EAR
CHAKRA
TE 17

KEY POINT
TE 4

GALL BLADDER
MERIDIAN

ANTERIOR
HEART
CHAKRA
CON 17

TRIPLE ENERGIZER
MERIDIAN

POSTERIOR
HEART
CHAKRA
GOV 10

ASSOCIATIONS

Major Chakra : Heart

INTERCOSTAL
CHAKRA
SP 21

Meridians : Gall Bladder
Triple Energizer

INTERCOSTAL
CHAKRA
SP 21

GALL BLADDER
MERIDIAN

Key Points : TE 4
GB 37

Color : Green

GALL BLADDER
MERIDIAN

Symptons : Eye Strain
Thoracic Pain & Stiffness
Diaphagmatic Pain
Head Shingles
Thoracic Shingles

KEY POINT
GB 37

KEY POINT
GB 37

FIGURE 1.17. *Associations of the Ear and Intercostal Chakras*

Local Symptoms

Local symptoms of the Ear chakra include localized ear-swelling, mas-toiditis, torticollis, tinnitus, mild deafness of traumatic etiology, otitis media, Bell's palsy, dizziness, and light-headedness.

General Symptoms

General symptoms of the Ear chakra include eye strain, cataract, thoracic pain, thoracic stiffness and joint pain, lower rib pain, diaphragmatic pain (or "side stitch"), and head shingles (herpes zoster).

INTERCOSTAL CHAKRA

The Intercostal chakra is situated in the mid-auxiliary line in the sixth intercostal space at acupoint SP 21. The Key point is GB 37 situated five cun superior to the lateral malleolus just anterior to the fibula.

Local Symptoms

Local symptoms include pain in the chest, discomfort in the chest, and intercostal shingles.

General Symptoms

The Intercostal chakra shares the same symptoms as the Ear chakra with the addition of general weakness and discomfort in the limbs (See Figure 1.17).

The practicalities of using the minor chakras will be discussed in Chapter Three and Chapter Four. Try to remember that chakras both major and minor are most effective when treated in combination with their coupled major and minor chakras.

COMBINATION OF MAJOR
AND MINOR CHAKRAS

Remember, the minor chakras do not have a gateway to the emotional body. Each, though, has a penetration to the more subtle edge of the etheric body which makes them more powerful than ordinary acupoints that are used for sedation and pain relief or even the eight key points of the extraordinary meridians and the "four gates" points. In clinical use, the major and minor chakras can be easily combined into treatment formula to give six very powerful modalities. When chakra combinations are used, the treatment of more chronic conditions is possible. To refresh your memory, the combinations are as follows:

1. The **Spleen** minor chakra is coupled with the **Sacral** and **Solar Plexus** major chakras.
2. The **Hand** and **Foot** minor chakras are coupled with the **Crown** major chakra.
3. The **Elbow** and **Knee** minor chakras are coupled with the **Base** major chakra.
4. The **Groin** and **Clavicular** minor chakras are coupled with the **Brow** major chakra.
5. The **Shoulder** and **Navel** minor chakras are coupled with the **Throat** major chakra.
6. The **Ear** and **Intercostal** minor chakras are coupled with the **Heart** major chakra.

SYMPTOMATOLOGY OF THE COMBINED CHAKRAS

The following lists represent the most common conditions treatable with chakra acupuncture.

CROWN, HAND, AND FOOT

Head shingles (herpes zoster), cervical spondylosis, metatarsalgia, chronic foot-related conditions, vertigo, hypertension, chronic headaches, and migraines.

BROW, GROIN, AND CLAVICLE

All chronic respiratory disease, throat conditions, migraine, catarrh, general infectious disease, altered hearing, some chronic genitourinary conditions, and chronic lower back pain.

THROAT, SHOULDER, AND NAVEL

Asthma, colitis, irritable bowel syndrome, frozen shoulder, chronic sinusitis, and introversion.

HEART, EAR, AND INTERCOSTAL

Thoracic herpes, facial neuralgia, generalized heart conditions, circulatory conditions, palpitation, varicosities, benign tumors, growths, and cysts.

SOLAR PLEXUS, SACRAL, AND SPLEEN

Conditions of the auto-immune system, glandular fever, chronic fatigue syndrome or myalgic encephalomyelitis (ME), depression, worry, eczema, hay fever, lymphatic obstruction, menopausal irregularity, menstrual irregularity, impotence, some symptoms of rheumatoid arthritis, edema, and water retention.

BASE, ELBOW, AND KNEE

Chronic spinal conditions, ankylosing spondylitis, lumbar spine arthritis, chronic lower back pain, elbow and knee arthritis, chronic cystitis, chronic nephritis, lethargy, depression, bone-related conditions, and fractures—useful especially when idiopathic or when encouraging a bone to heal at a faster rate.

As you can see, many more chronic conditions may be addressed using chakra combinations than by treating just one chakra in isolation. Do not forget that by treating the chakras, you are treating the *cause* of the condition.

TRADITIONAL CHINESE MEDICINE
AND THE CHAKRAS

As you might know, the chakra energy system stems from a different heritage than Traditional Chinese Medicine (TCM). Chapter Two covers the various similarities and differences of these two medical practices, but shows how we, as practitioners, may use the two philosophies together to the benefit of our patients. In this chapter, you will learn how TCM diagnosis and analysis may be used to ascertain chakra imbalance and how by balancing and treating the chakra energies we can create a whole new paradigm of medicine that truly combines these two systems of traditional medicine. It is thought that the roots of chakra energy philosophy lie within the Indian Ayurvedic system of medicine. Though there are many types of traditional medicine—each based on a different philosophy, each one emphasizes a *vital force* in one way or another. Ayurvedic medicine calls its vital force *prana,* as do traditional Tibetan and Japanese medicine. In TCM, vital force is called *chi.* Ayurvedic medicine is not the only tradition from which chakra energy system philosophy evolved. Many traditional approaches to medicine have influenced the development of the chakra energy system. Traditional Tibetan, Buddhist, and Vietnamese texts all contribute to what we now consider to be the chakras. There is such an amazing wealth of material in alternative medicine that has been handed down through the generations over the last two millennia that it remains a humbling experience on my part to attempt to portray these philosophies to the twenty-first century reader.

AYURVEDIC MEDICINE

Ayurvedic medicine is said to have originated from the ancient Hindu texts, the Vedas. The word *ayus* means "life" and *veda* means "knowledge." Most scholars now believe that Ayurveda was born out of a union of Hindu and Buddhist traditions. To quote *The Healing Path* by Jacqueline Young, "The body is seen as a microcosmic universe in which the five great primordial elements *(panchamahabhutas)*—ether *(akasha)*, air *(vayu)*, fire *(agni)*, water *(jala)*, and earth *(prithvi)*—combine to form three humors *(doshas)* known as wind *(vata)*, choler *(pitta)*, and phlegm *(kapha)*. Each dosha has its own qualities and functions in relation to the body. The balance between these doshas determines individual constitution *(prakriti)* and predisposition to disease. Constitution is also affected by the strength of a person's "digestive fire" *(agni)* and bowel function *(kostha)*. Seven tissues *(dhatus)* and their waste products *(malas)* make up the physical body and a network of channels circulate fluids and essences around the body. Disease occurs if lifestyle, mental, or external factors cause an imbalance in one or more of these components" (2002).

DIAGNOSIS AND TREATMENT

An eight fold approach is typically used in Ayurvedic diagnosis, involving the pulse, tongue, voice, skin texture, vision, general appearance, urine, and stool. The information gleaned from the examination of these facets is combined with information about a person's constitution, age, body type, and astrological alignment (which detects karma and ancestral qualities). Treatment aims to restore the energy balance of the *doshas* using a combination of herbal medicine, massage, physical manipulation, and diet. There are also five *panchakarma* purification techniques used for cleansing and detoxifying the body. On the surface, there seems to be a similarity in the diagnosis and treatment between Ayurvedic medicine and TCM. When it comes to the esoteric energy *concepts,* however, there is quite a different approach.

ENERGY CONCEPTS—
NADIS, SUSHUMNA, IDA, AND PINGALA

It is said that the Etheric aura is filled with thousands of energy channels called *nadis* through which vital force *(prana)* flows. Through this extensive network of subtle channels the chakras connect to the physical body. Congestion of the *nadis* with stagnant energy (either from in to out or out to in) affects the Physical Body, which then exhibits symptoms of disorder. Richard Gerber, MD, in his book *Vibrational Medicine* states, "The *nadis* are formed by fine threads of subtle energy matter. They are different from meridians, which actually have a physical counterpart in the meridian duct system. The *nadis* represent an extensive network of fluid-like energies which parallel the bodily nerves in their abundance. In the Eastern yogic literature, the chakras have been metaphorically visualized as flowers. The *nadis* are symbolic of the petals and fine roots of the flowerlike chakras that distribute the *prana* of each chakra into the physical body. Various sources have described up to 72,000 *nadis* or Etheric channels of energy in the subtle anatomy of humans. These unique channels are interwoven with the physical nervous system. Because of this intricate interconnection with the nervous system, the *nadis* affect the nature and quality of nerve transmission within the extensive network of the brain, spinal cord, and peripheral nerves" (1988).

There are also three main components of the *nadis* that are aligned on the vertical axis of the trunk (anterior and posterior) from the Crown to the Base chakras—these being the *Sushumna, Ida,* and *Pingala.* Most traditional texts agree that the *Sushumna nadi* is only situated along the spinal cord—the main channel for the flow of nervous energy up and down the spine. From the *Sushumna nadi,* thousands of minor *nadis* branch out and link with the nervous system of the physical body. In my experience, I have found the *Sushumna nadi* to be situated (and therefore represented) on the anterior aspect of the trunk as well: thus, we may equate its dorsal aspect to the *Du Mai* (Governor channel) and the anterior aspect to the *Ren Mai* (Conception channel). The *Ida nadi* is aligned on the left side of the spine and the *Pingala Nadi* on the right.

As discussed in Chapter One, at the Etheric level, a major chakra is formed where twenty-one *nadis* intersect and a minor chakra where fourteen *nadis* cross. In TCM, *Ida* would be interpreted as *yin* and *Pingala* would be seen as *yang* energy. Many texts give the three main *nadi* a spinal connotation, whereas my research indicates both anterior and posterior locations and thus both anterior and posterior chakras. The anterior *(yin)* aspect may be used in chronic, emotional, and organic conditions and the spinal aspects *(yang)* are mostly used in musculo-skeletal conditions. Due to the differing interpretations *Sushumna, Ida,* and *Pingala nadi,* they have different anatomical connotations depending on the culture from where they originated.

Traditional Indian (Ayurvedic), Indonesian, and Tibetan medicine have the coiled serpent *(caduceus)* approach, whereas traditional Buddhist philosophy (including Japanese, Burmese, and Vietnamese) shows that the *Sushumna nadi* flows along the spinal cord and that the *Ida* and *Pingala* flow in relatively straight lines that are parallel to the *Sushumna*. In the latter case the *Ida* and *Pingala* represent the Bladder meridian (inner and outer aspects) alongside the spine and the Kidney and Stomach meridians (equivalent inner and outer aspects), alongside the Conception meridian and the *Sushumna* the Governor *(Du Mai)* and the Conception *(Ren mai)* channels. Figure 2.1 shows a diagrammatic representation of the Conception, Stomach, and Kidney meridians on the anterior aspect of the trunk and the Governor and Inner and Outer Bladder meridians on the posterior aspect. Figure 2.2 shows one interpretation of the *Sushumna, Ida,* and *Pingala nadi* which very closely mimic the TCM interpretation. The "crossing over" aspect (see Figure 2.3) resembles the medical emblem of the Caduceus or the coiled serpent. *Ida* is associated with coolness, the moon, the right brain hemisphere, and the parasympathetic nervous system, whereas *Pingala* is associated with the sun, heat, the left brain hemisphere, and the sympathetic nervous system.

See page 99, Figure 2.1. Diagrammatic Representation of the Conception, Governor, Stomach, Kidney, and Bladder Meridians; page 100, Figure 2.2. Representation of the *Sushumna, Ida,* and *Pingala Nadis* (One); and page 101, Figure 2.3. Representation of the *Sushumna, Ida,* and *Pingala Nadis* (Two).

I am not "on the fence" about these opposing approaches. I simply believe that they can *both* be correct. We are, after all, dealing with subtle esoteric energy systems, and the fact remains that no single system of medicine ever has a monopoly on the truth. I concur with the theory that there is a crossover of *Ida* and *Pingala* energies at the five diaphragmatic areas of the body, creating the archetypal chakra formation, though notably the *Ida* and *Pingala* energies also link with the Kidney and Bladder channels.

Note, the five diaphragmatic regions of the body are the sphenoid (Brow chakra), thoracic inlet (Throat chakra), thoracic outlet (Heart chakra), diaphragm (Solar Plexus chakra), and the pelvic diaphragm (Sacral chakra). The five diaphragmatic intersections explain how at each chakra level there is a dominant endocrine, autonomic nerve, and nerve plexus association, while at the same time the "energies" may be "felt" flowing along the vertical axis. Though demonstrated in acupuncture by the *de qui* response, this energy is more easily felt through the application of acupressure or craniosacral therapy. My experience working with patients leads me to believe that the *Sushumna nadi* energy flow equates to the flow of the cerebro-spinal fluid at the spinal level (conception energy flow at the anterior aspect). This theory also explains the highly effective "associated effect" or "back transporting" points along the inner and outer aspects of the bladder meridian that are energetically linked to internal organs by internal pathways (also called reflected pathways or "reflexes," as in reflexology). There is also an organic link on the front of the torso by the *hara* or abdominal reflex areas that are also linked with the *Sushumna, Ida,* and *Pingala* nadi and chakras. In my experience, whether the links are energetic, reflected, trigger, or nervous system does not matter! I have spent a quarter of a century attempting to figure this one out and still have not made any conclusive or rational decisions. It is what it is.

REMAINING NADIS ENERGY CHANNELS

In *Theories of the Chakras: Bridge to Higher Consciousness* Dr. Hiroshi Motoyama writes about the remaining *nadi* in some detail (1981). I was privileged to attend one of his seminars in London in 1985 when he spoke on this subject. Motoyama claims that there are fifteen other major *nadi* that often have correlations with TCM meridians, either the eight extra-ordinary channels, the main meridians (stomach, gall bladder and kidney), or the distinct meridians. Where the other 72,000 *nadi* are situated is immaterial. When dealing with the Physical-Etheric or the Etheric-Emotional auras, we only have the word of "all seeing" clairvoyants to guide us. How the figure of 72,000 was discovered boggles the mind. It suffices to say, the Etheric Body consists of a "pea soup" of whirling energies called the *nadis* that intercommunicate with the physical body via the chakras. Knowledge of the *nadis* is vital and remains one of the cornerstone principles of energy medicine—especially in the practice of traditional acupuncture.

AYURVEDIC AND TRADITIONAL CHINESE MEDICINE

Correlations abound between traditional Indian medicine (Ayurvedic) and TCM from acupoints, to meridians, to the eight extra-ordinary meridians, to Key points, to the six *Chious,* to the Law of Five Elements. In this chapter, we will discuss the correlations then discuss the areas of analysis and diagnosis of the tongue, pulse, abdomen, and the concept of tender points.

ACUPOINTS

The research proving the existence of acupoints is extensive. Thousands of trials and experiments have concluded that they actually *do* exist. Scientifically measured, they are points on the body's skin that show a lower electrical resistance to that of the surrounding tissues. This analysis does not just include acupoints that lie on the meridians but non-meridian acupoints as well. My theory is that there is no actual difference between acupoints and body reflex points—this theory will be fully explored in a future book tentatively entitled—*Light Touch Reflextherapy.* Scientific analysis tells us that acupoints may be likened to minute micro-fibril bundles of connective tissue that in some way are connected with the central nervous system. The trained finger can actually feel these points in that they are usually tender when they are in need of treatment. It is thought that each acupoint represents a "micro-chakra" in that they can be considered as "energy vortices" that draw *chi (prana)* into or out of the body's energy flow and provide access points whereby the *chi* flow of the body can be directly influenced by these vortices. If you can think of these acupoints as tiny energy vortices, then you can easily understand how major energy vortices of the body (major and minor chakras) have a corresponding physical component or acupoint. When the chakras were considered only as part of the domain of yoga and meditation, it was assumed that they were gateways of spiritual energy situated within the subtle bodies without physical counterparts. This is not true. The physical body is as much a part of our energetic being as the other six layers and should be considered as such. It is extremely important to understand that when you needle an acupoint you are not only affecting the symptomatology of the physical body but the remaining subtle bodies as well.

Meridians

If acupoints have been scientifically proven to exist and work by manipulating the central nervous system (brain and spinal cord), what about the meridians on which the acupoints are situated? Meridians have not yet been researched enough by Western scientists, but the lack of scientific data does not negate the existence and usefulness of meridians. In ancient times there was no knowledge of the central nervous system, and the brain was not considered to have any affect on the internal organs. At this time Western medical practitioners may recognize acupuncture as a proven healthcare method without the knowledge of meridians, but nevertheless treatment using the traditional meridians does work! Slowly but surely science is catching up to Eastern medicine, and some gifted scientists are studying how traditional meridians work as energy channels. James Oschman, PhD, considers meridians to be demonstrable low-resistance, bio-physical pathways as he describes in his book *Energy Medicine in Therapeutics and Human Performance* (2003). Thomas Myers considers meridians to be like "anatomy trains" which are linkages of fascia and bone that wind through the body, connecting head to toe and core to periphery, as he describes in *Anatomy Trains—Myofascial Meridians for Manual and Movement Therapists* (2001).

Gone are the days when we thought of meridians as actual physical tubes or canals that house *chi*. We now consider meridians to be a part of the energy matrix linked to the central nervous system. The energy matrix, a very powerful system of energy channels, can easily be treated together with the chakra energy system as a complementary or back-up system. The meridians may be stroked with the flow of energy as pre-treatment to the chakra treatment or stimulated at the Source point as part of the chakra treatment. I took a considerable amount of time to research the definitive correlations between the chakras and meridians. I have now used these associated pathways for twenty-five years, and I have verified them in treatment. To remind you, they are as follows.

TABLE 2.1. ASSOCIATION OF THE MAJOR AND MINOR CHAKRAS WITH MERIDIANS

Chakra	Meridian(s)
Crown	Triple Energizer
Brow	Gall Bladder and Yangwei Mai
Throat	Lung, Large Intestine and Yangchiao Mai
Heart	Heart, Small Intestine and Yinwei Mai
Solar Plexus	Liver, Stomach and Dai Mai
Sacral	Pericardium, Spleen and Yinchiao Mai
Base	Kidney, Bladder, Governor, Conception and Chong mai
Spleen	Spleen and Lung
Foot	Kidney
Hand	Heart
Knee	Bladder
Elbow	Small Intestine
Groin	Liver
Clavicular	Pericardium

Chakra	Meridian(s)
Shoulder	Large Intestine
Navel	Stomach
Intercostal	Triple Energizer
Ear	Gall Bladder

The meridian back-up system is generally used in the treatment of chronic conditions. The Base chakra is associated with five meridians including three of the extra meridians, explaining the Base chakra's power in the treatment of chronic maladies. In Chapter Four, I discuss practical methods of treating the Base chakra.

THE EIGHT EXTRAORDINARY MERIDIANS

As every traditional acupuncturist knows, the eight extraordinary meridians and the knowledge of their Key points can be extremely useful tools in energy balancing. Traditional acupuncturists use these points and channels every day and understand their importance. I personally know three acupuncturists who *only* use these points in virtually every condition. To remind you, the eight extra meridians are:

1. *Du Mai* (Governor) channel—Key point SI 3
2. *Ren Mai* (Conception) channel—Key point LU 7
3. *Chong Mai* (Vital) channel—Key point SP 4
4. *Dai Mai* (Belt or Girdle) channel—Key point GB 41
5. *Yangchiao Mai* (*Yang* Motility) channel—Key point BL 62
6. *Yinchiao Mai* (*Yin* Motility) channel—Key point KID 6
7. *Yangwei Mai* (*Yang* Regulator) channel—Key point TE 5
8. *Yinwei Mai* (*Yin* Regulator) channel—Key point PC 6

As Table 2.1 shows, each of the extra meridians is also associated with a chakra. The knowledge of associated extra meridians gives an extra dimension to your treatment of the chakras: the practicalities of meridian use will be fully discussed in Chapter Four. Several years ago I gave some thought to the commonly held (but esoteric) idea of chakras being active and receptive at certain times of our lives. This means that during each span of seven years of our lives a particular chakra resonates more than the others, in a similar way that each organ has a heightened energy level for two hours during the day (Chinese Clock).

With each of the "seven ages of man" a different chakra is highlighted. The more open and active chakra still resonates after its seventh year of heightened energy but not as much as the newly predominant chakra. The heightened chakra may cause certain imbalances and conditions or it may be beneficial—it depends on the general constitution of the body. Traditional wisdom indicates that the Base chakra is associated with our ancestry and genetic coding—in other words, we are born with a hereditary blueprint of energy make-up at conception (I will not be discussing potential karmic influences here). The Sacral chakra is then "opened" and starts to resonate from the birth to the age of seven. Between the ages of eight to fourteen the Solar Plexus is highlighted—this is when we would be affected by childhood diseases such as glandular fever or the start of allergic reactions. Then between the ages of fifteen to twenty-two we are drawn toward the opposite sex and have "affairs of the heart." The Throat chakra is highlighted between the ages of twenty-two and twenty-eight. Intuitional prowess may occur between age twenty-nine and thirty-five. We reach the peak of our given profession and reasoning powers with the Crown chakra highlighted between ages thirty-six to forty-two. The Throat chakra is again highlighted between the ages fifty to fifty-six when we tend to get problems with the bowel and eliminative system. The Heart center is once again highlighted between ages fifty-seven to sixty-three when people tend to have circulatory and heart conditions. The Sacral chakra commences to resonate again close to the biblical "three score years and ten" when we then enter our "second childhood" through activation of the Base chakra.

The highlighted periods of chakra strength may be viewed as esoteric mumbo jumbo or as knowledge that can guide to our acupuncture treatments. If we know the constitution (through the Case History) and age of the patient, even if we do nothing else, balancing the associated chakra (with its Key points) and the associated extraordinary meridian (with its Key points) can be very useful. I have used this balancing method hundreds of times with amazing results. Following the table below are listed a few symptoms that we can expect to meet at these times that are associated with imbalance to the chakra and its related extraordinary meridian.

TABLE 2.2. ASSOCIATION OF CHAKRAS, KEY POINTS, EXTRA MERIDIANS AND ENERGY PEAK

Chakra	Chakra Key Points	Extraordinary Meridian(s)	Meridian Key Points	Energy Peak Age
Crown	Con 4 TE 5	—	—	36–42
Brow	Gov 4 SP 6	Yangwei Mai	TE 5	29–35 and 43–49
Throat	Con 6 LR 5	Yangchiao Mai	BL 62	22–28 and 50–56
Heart	Gov 7 HT 1	Yinwei Mai	PC 6	15–21 and 57–63
Solar Plexus	Con 17 TE 4	Dai Mai	GB 41	8–14 and 64–70
Sacral	Gov 12 PC 3	Yinchiao Mai	KID 6	Birth–7 and 71–77
Base	Con 22 LR 8	Du Ma Ren Mai Chong Mai	SI 3 LU 7 SP 4	Ancestral and 78+

SYMPTOMATOLOGY OF THE ABOVE CHAKRAS

- **Crown**—Headache, dizziness, vertigo, shock.
- **Brow** or *Yangwei Mai*—Aversion to cold, fever, acute febrile disease, cerebrospinal fluid (CSF) imbalances, hormonal imbalances, headache.

- **Throat** or *Yangchiao Mai*—Respiratory and skin conditions, coordination and muscular movement of lower limbs, insomnia.
- **Heart** or *Yinwei Mai*—Circulatory conditions, emotions, chest pains, angina, asthma.
- **Solar Plexus** or *Dai Mai*—Digestive conditions, lumbar weakness.
- **Sacral** or *Yinchiao Mai*—Urinary conditions, water imbalance, lower limb weakness.
- **Base,** *Du Mai, Ren Mai, Chong Mai*—All chronic spinal conditions, hereditary conditions, arthritis, menopausal conditions, strong mental picture, severe depression.

KEY POINTS

When first contemplating using the chakra energy system with acupuncture over twenty-five years ago it seemed logical to me that some type of "access" point would be required just as the eight extraordinary meridians required a key to open the energy door. Using a Key point is not necessary when using this system of therapy with acupressure and healing as the chakra centers may be contacted, balanced, and treated directly without any other points being used. In *Healing with the Chakra Energy System,* I promulgated the use of the Key points when using acupressure solely as an added refinement to chakra treatment—it is not essential to the efficacy of the treatment. When using acupuncture, however, it *is essential* that Key points are used. Researching the Key points was the most difficult thing I had to do on my quest to perfect this therapy. They were arrived at as a combination of common sense, dowsing, guesswork, and trial-and-error on my poor unsuspecting patients. There are two Key points for each major chakra and one for each minor chakra. They are to be needled and stimulated prior to the chakra acupoints being needled—practical applications appear in Chapter Three and Chapter Four.

THE SIX CHIOUS

The Six *Chious* represent logical meridian combinations of the twelve meridians into six units. The pairs of meridians also describe layers of energy in the body ranging from superficial *yang* to deepest *yin*. They are, from the most superficial to the deepest energies:

- Small Intestine and Bladder—*Tai Yang* or Great *Yang,*
- Triple Energizer and Gall Bladder—*Chao Yang* or Lesser *Yang,*
- Large Intestine and Stomach—*Yang Ming* or Bright *Yang,*
- Lung and Spleen—*Tai Yin* or Great *Yin,*
- Pericardium and Liver—*Tsui Yin* or Decreasing *Yin,*
- Heart and Kidney—*Chao Yin* or Lesser *Yin.*

From this list, it can be seen that each combination of meridians may be viewed as *one* single meridian each one representing an ever deepening of the body's energies. In practical treatment terms, the *Chious* are useful in the treatment of "invading" or "perverse" energy called *fong, thap,* or *hua.* The weather system held much importance in ancient China in that it was held responsible for many ailments. The list below adds the weather systems and which meridians would be affected. If the superficial meridians are not treated within a certain time span, the perverse energy will be driven deeper into the constitution to affect another *Chiou*—and so on.

- SI and BL—*Tai Yang*—Heat and Cold
- TE and GB—*Chao Yang*—Heat and Wind
- LI and ST—*Yang Ming*—Dryness and Humidity
- LU and SP—*Tai Yin*—Dryness and Humidity
- PC and LR—*Tsui Yin*—Heat and Wind
- HT and KI—*Chao Yin*—Heat and Cold

Visibly, the system of Heat and Cold (each in excess) may open a pathway for invading *fong* energy into the system. Once the constitution is in a weakened state, the same weather system also affects the deepest energies.

The philosophy of the six *Chious* may be translated to include the chakra energy system. As you can see below, each meridian combination traverses several major and minor chakras which may be useful in analysis and treatment. Even if a meridian does not travel through a particular acupoint, an area of influence exists around each point that will affect the meridian flow. Distinct and inner pathways of the meridians must also be taken into account. The energy flow of the six *Chious* is as follows:

TAI YANG

- **Small Intestine (SI).** Energy flows from Hand chakra to Elbow chakra to Shoulder chakra to posterior Throat chakra to anterior Brow chakra.
- **Bladder (BL).** Energy flows from anterior Brow chakra to posterior Throat chakra to posterior Heart chakra to posterior Solar Plexus chakra to posterior Sacral chakra to posterior Base chakra to Knee chakra to Foot chakra.

This energy system flows from the hand to the foot with a cross over at the Brow chakra and is the most superficial of the body's energies.

CHAO YANG

- **Gall Bladder (GB).** Energy flows from Foot chakra to Knee chakra to Groin chakra to Intercostal chakra to Shoulder chakra to Ear chakra to anterior Brow chakra.
- **Triple Energizer (TE).** Energy flows from anterior Brow chakra to Ear chakra to Shoulder chakra to Elbow chakra to Hand chakra.

This energy system flows from the foot to the hand with a cross over at the Brow chakra and is a deeper energy continuation of the *Tai Yang*.

YANG MING

- **Large Intestine (LI).** Energy flows from Hand chakra to Elbow chakra to Shoulder chakra to posterior Throat chakra to anterior Brow chakra.
- **Stomach (ST).** Energy flows from anterior Brow chakra to anterior Throat chakra to Clavicular chakra to Navel chakra to Groin chakra to Knee chakra to Foot chakra.

This energy system flows from the hand to the foot with a cross over at the Brow chakra and is a deeper energy continuation of the *Chao Yang*.

TAI YIN

- **Spleen (SP).** Energy flows from Foot chakra to Knee chakra to Groin chakra to Intercostal chakra to anterior Throat chakra.
- **Lung (LU).** Energy flows from anterior Throat chakra to Shoulder chakra to Elbow chakra to Hand chakra.

This energy system flows from the foot to the hand with a cross over at the anterior Throat chakra and is a deeper energy continuation of the *Yang Ming*.

TSUI YIN

- **Pericardium (PC).** Energy flows from Hand chakra to Elbow chakra to Shoulder chakra to anterior Throat chakra.
- **Liver (LR).** Energy flows from anterior Throat chakra to Intercostal chakra to Groin chakra to Knee chakra to Foot chakra.

This energy system flows from the hand to the foot with a cross over at the Throat chakra and is a deeper energy continuation of *Tai Yin*.

CHAO YIN

- **Kidney (KID).** Energy flows from Foot chakra to Knee chakra to Groin chakra to anterior Base chakra to Navel chakra to anterior Sacral chakra to anterior Solar Plexus chakra to anterior Heart chakra to Intercostal chakra to anterior Throat chakra.
- **Heart (HT).** Energy flows from anterior Throat chakra to anterior Heart chakra to Shoulder chakra to Elbow chakra to Hand chakra.

This energy system flows from the foot to the hand with a cross over at the Throat chakra and is a deeper energy continuation of *Tsui Yin*. It represents the deepest of the body's energies.

The following conclusions may be drawn from a basic knowledge of the meridian pathways:

- The three yang *Chious* each have an energetic crossover between component meridians at the Brow chakra. Also, the three *yin Chious* each cross at the Throat chakra. Therefore, the more superficial energetic treatment is geared toward the higher frequency of the Brow chakra and the deeper energetic treatment requires treatment via the lower frequency of the Throat chakra (Please remember that the *Chious* mostly deal with weather invasions and not viruses—where the Throat chakra would be used primarily).

- In order to reverse the effects of perverse energy at a particular level, the associated chakra level is used together with the *Tsing* points for the *yang Chious* and the *Luo* acupoints points for the *yin Chious*. The *Tsing* or "nail" points are at the end of the meridian and the *Luo* points represent the communication between the constituent meridians of the *Chiou*.

- Experience has shown that copper and zinc needles are more beneficial when used in the three *yang Chious* and ordinary stainless steel with the *yin Chious*. If you do not possess copper and zinc needles then ordinary stainless steel needles will suffice. The altered metal needle treatments will be discussed in Appendix One.

Here are appropriate treatment rationales for each of the *Chious:*

TAI YANG

- *Symptoms* include fever, perspiration, thirst, headaches, and fear of cold.

- *Treatment*—*Yintang*—BL 67—SI 1 (copper on the *Tsing* points and zinc on the Brow chakra).

CHAO YANG

- *Symptoms*—Fever, shivering, vomiting, nausea, bitter mouth, and rapid pulse.

- *Treatment*—*Yintang*—TE 1—GB 44 (copper on the *Tsing* points and zinc on the Brow chakra).

YANG MING

- *Symptoms*—Diarrhea, perspiration, thirst, anxiety, high fever, and fear of heat.
- *Treatment*—*Yintang*—ST 45—LI 1 (copper on the *Tsing* points and zinc on the Brow chakra).

TAI YIN

- *Symptoms*—Cold, shivering, heavy yellow coating on tongue, abdominal distension, vomiting, diarrhea, no thirst, pulse—slow and thin.
- *Treatment*—Con 22—LU 7—SP 4.

TSUI YIN

- *Symptoms*—Diarrhea, vomiting, limbs cold, weak pulse, thirst, pains in chest, shivering, and fever.
- *Treatment*—Con 22—PC 6—LR 5.

CHAO YIN

- *Symptoms*—Cold throughout the body, icy cold limbs, fear of the cold, fatigue, weak pulse, feeling of fullness in the chest, and restlessness.
- *Treatment*—Con 22—HT 5—KID 4.

THE LAW OF FIVE TRANSFORMATIONS (ELEMENTS)

Traditionally trained acupuncturists do not need to be told of the beauty, complexity, and awe-inspiring significance of the Law of Five Elements. Anyone who has had the fortune to be able to learn (or better still to teach it) has entered a world of untold treasures. It is a law that explains the intricacies of both TCM and many other traditional approaches to medicine. I well remember being introduced to this law in 1976 on my Licentiate of Acupuncture course in London. All I had wanted to do before the course was to be able to stick needles in patients without necessarily understanding the philosophy behind acupuncture. My whole world was subsequently transformed by the intricate philosophy that was explained to me. It is said that no one can ever know too much about it. There are some practitioners who would say that true acupuncture does not exist without usage of the Law of Five Elements. Western trained acupuncturists and those who only learn and practice symptomatic pain relief have missed out on the crown jewel of acupuncture. There is *no way* that I can improve on the Law of Five Elements, but I want to show you how it may be made even more exciting by incorporating the chakra energy system.

Here I will summarize the Law of Five Elements for those who are not familiar with it already. The philosophy of TCM is based on Taoism which is involved with observations of the natural world and the manner in which it operates. The human body, which is part of the natural world, may be viewed as dynamic energy consisting of organs (either *yin* or *yang*) that have an interchange with each other based on what occurs in nature. The Chinese observed that everywhere in nature there is dynamic interchange and that the human body is no exception. Each organ (including the Triple Energizer and Pericardium) is placed in one of five elements. The *Yang* organs are on the outside, representing the superficial. The *Yin* organs are on the inside, representing the inner economy. The five elements are not chemical elements but rather five aspects of nature representing the rhythms of life. They are represented as Fire, Earth, Metal, Water, and Wood.

There are three ways of viewing the energy link of the elements. In the Law of Five Elements, there are cycles. The *Sheng* or engendering cycle is the creative cycle. The *Ko* cycle is the controlling cycle. There is also the reverse *Ko* cycle. In the *Sheng* cycle, fire produces ashes (earth); earth (as ore) produces metal; metal (by hydrolysis) produces water; water produces wood (in the sense that water makes plant life possible); and wood produces fire (as in fuel). With the *Ko* cycle, fire subjugates metal (as in melting); metal subjugates wood (as in chopping or cutting); wood subjugates earth (by penetrating it with roots); earth subjugates water (by absorbing it or providing a dam or obstruction); and water subjugates fire (by extinguishing it).

See Figures 2. 4 and 2.5 and the table below for easy reference of the Five Elements.

TABLE 2.3 THE LAW OF THE FIVE TRANSFORMATIONS (ELEMENTS)

Element	Fire	Earth	Metal	Water	Wood
Direction	South	Center	West	North	East
Color	Red	Yellow	White	Blue/Black	Green
System	Circulation	Connective	Skin	Bones	Muscles Tendons
Sense	Speech	Taste	Smell	Hearing	Sight
Facial	Mouth	Tongue	Nose	Ears	Eyes
Emotion	Joy	Sympathy	Grief	Fear	Anger
Season	Summer	Late Summer	Autumn (Fall)	Winter	Spring
Weather	Heat	Humidity	Dryness	Cold	Wind
Taste	Bitter	Sweet	Pungent	Putrid	Sour
Yin Organ (Zang)	Heart	Spleen	Lung	Kidney	Liver
Yang organ (Fu)	Small Intestine	Stomach	Large Intestine	Bladder	Gall Bladder

Examples of clinical importance:

• Patients can sometimes be archetyped according to which system and part of the body is affected. For example, a person suffering from irritable bowel syndrome (IBS) has pale skin, suffers from catarrh, and feels worse in the autumn and in dry weather—he or she would be archetyped as a "metal" person.

- *Chi* energy can be transferred from element to element, thus providing a balance of energy within the body. The Tonification points are used to balance energy via the *Sheng* cycle either around the *yang* organs or *yin* organs.

- By taking a correct case history, you will be able to ascertain how the patients conditions have occurred, one following on from the other. The process of disease progression and symptom formation that occurs within the body is seemingly random but actually follows, in a logical sequence, the Law of Five Elements. Vital Force improves health but Disease Force works against Vital Force. Once disease has entered the body (often at infancy), Disease Force or destructive force rampages its way from organ to organ in a reverse *Ko* manner. Reverse *Ko* disease formation often occurs within the *Yang* organs. When illness is superficial, i.e., on the *Yang* cycle, this means that disease proceeds from the large intestine to the small intestine, to the bladder, to the stomach, to the gall bladder, and completes the cycle back at the large bowel. Once Disease Force enters the *Yin* system, the illness is much deeper and life threatening. Disease force can travel from, for example, the spleen to the liver, to the lung, to the heart, to the kidney, and completes the cycle at the spleen again. Many treatments could be tried along the way, and if they were allopathic in nature could be suppressive. Many experts agree that allopathic medicine can hasten the progression of Disease Force. Natural medicine, including acupuncture, would halt the progression of Disease Force and would enable the body to fight by using its own vital force. Take a closer look at some of your patients with attention to their particular histories and you may see them in a new light.

For example, imagine someone who has suffered a stroke with resultant painful spasms of the arms and legs. You question him or her. The summer heat is making the pain and discomfort worse. He or she has speech problems, a bitter taste in the mouth, and a ruddy complexion. Therefore, you can deduce that he or she is a Fire person. To be a Fire person means that the organs that comprise the Fire element—heart, small intestine, pericardium and triple energizer—need to be treated. The liver and gallbladder organs of the Wood element also need to be stimulated as they are the mother of the organs of the Fire element. It is useless to give localized therapy symptomatically if the general *chi* energy has not been addressed.

LAW OF FIVE ELEMENTS AND THE CHAKRA ENERGY SYSTEM

I would not be so bold as to claim to be able to improve the Law of Five Elements. What I can do, however, is to translate an understanding of the TCM basis of the Law into the language of the chakra energy system. In this way, the two knowledge bases can be used together. I hope that you will find this helpful.

(See page 102, Figure 2.4. Law of Five Elements—TCM and Figure 2.5. Law of Five Elements—Chakras.)

The real stumbling block when using the two systems in correlation with one another is the differing use of color with which the elements are traditionally associated. The colors are generally considered to be Fire— Red, Earth—Yellow, Metal—White, Water—Blue or Black, and Wood— Green. It remains, therefore, a great temptation to use the same colors with the chakras which is both misleading and impossible. Instead, reference the associated organs and systems that are linked with the relevant chakras. Figure 2.4 shows the traditional viewpoint of the Law of Five Elements with the colors usually prescribed. Figure 2.5 shows how it may be considered as part of the chakra system of healing, showing the colors associated with the chakras. Each element consists of the same internal organs as before. The *Sheng* and *Ko* cycles remain unchanged. Within the Fire element, the small intestine and triple energizer are associated with the Heart chakra, and the heart and pericardium are linked with the Crown chakra. Within the Earth element, the stomach is associated with the Solar Plexus chakra, and the spleen is linked with the Sacral chakra. The Metal element (lung and large intestine) is linked with the Throat chakra. The Water element (kidney and bladder) is linked with the Base chakra. The Wood element (liver and gall bladder) is linked with the Brow chakra.

What advantage to the patient does using the Law of Five elements add? Simply, adding a new dimension to a treatment enhances understanding of the patient and in this way enables the practitioner to analyze and to treat patients in a much more profound way. The added dimension of chakra energy in a treatment allows the practitioner to ascertain the *emotional, personality,* and *character* aspects of the patient that are associated with the individual organ, system, or meridian—not *just* the physical aspect that is treated under the Law without the knowledge of chakras.

To review, the associated emotional and mental aspects of the chakras are as follows:

- **Crown chakra**—Melancholy, phobias, delusion, illusion, pride, arrogance, and spiritual awareness.
- **Brow chakra**—Anger, rage, indecision, indifference, lack of moral courage, changeable, and discontentment.
- **Throat chakra**—Shyness, introversion, paranoia, insecurity, suppressed emotions, agoraphobia, lack of expression, and inability to change direction.
- **Heart chakra**—Tearfulness, anxiety, depression, detachedness, euphoria, self-pity, and inability to show or receive love.
- **Solar Plexus chakra**—Depression (deeper than Heart), anxiety, pity, panic, claustrophobia, reluctance to change, and rigid thoughts and belief systems.
- **Sacral chakra**—Envy, jealousy, lust, promiscuity, low self-esteem, and poor communication.
- **Base chakra**—Insecurity, doubt, severe phobias, mind in turmoil, fear of change, loneliness, and inability to ground oneself.

A patient might visit you for the first time with an emotional condition but would be likely to wait until your second session when confidence has been earned to divulge personal information regarding emotional issues. Though sometimes overlooked, in fact, the clinical significance of emotional etiology is often more important than physical etiology. Therefore at any stage of the treatment (as the main thrust or final energy balancing), apply the following method:

1. Ascertain correct chakra imbalance by taking a thorough case history.
2. Follow diagnostic and analytical methods using specific directions found in Chapter Three and Chapter Four.
3. Needle the Source point of the element at the same time as the anterior chakra point. These are the Source and anterior chakra points for each of the main chakras:
   - Crown chakra—Gov 20 with HT 7 and PC 7.
   - Brow chakra—Extra 1 *(Yintang)* with LR 3 and GB 40.
   - Throat chakra—Con 22 with LU 9 and LI 4.
   - Heart chakra—Con 17 with SI 3 and TE 4.
   - Solar Plexus chakra—Con 14 with ST 42.
   - Sacral chakra—Con 6 with SP 3.
   - Base chakra—Con 2 with KID 3 and BL 64.

   These points would be treated either in isolation or with other treatment schedules, depending on the condition and energy state (constitution) of the patient.
4. As the final energy balance of the treatment session, the Tonification points may be used. They are:
   - *Yin* cycle—SP 2 to LU 11 to KID 7 to LR 8 to either HT 7 or PC 9.
   - *Yang* cycle—ST 41 to LI 11 to BL 67 to GB 43 to either SI 3 or TE 3.

   Each point should be stimulated for a couple of seconds before withdrawal.

METHODS OF ANALYSIS

What methods of analysis and diagnosis do we have that enable us to draw conclusions as to which chakra to treat? They do not vary much from the tried and tested methods that are presently employed by TCM practitioners throughout the world. They are case history (question and answer), pulse diagnosis, tongue diagnosis, abdominal diagnosis, and tender acupoints. Other methods that were mentioned in my previous book, *Healing with the Chakra Energy System,* include using the hands in the Etheric Body to ascertain magnetic energy flow from the chakras, and using the Listening Posts on the occiput, skull, and heels. In addition to "hand dowsing," other forms of dowsing may be applied either with the hands or a pendulum. The analytical method of dowsing is very subjective and does not fall under the TCM umbrella. Another excellent method of analysis is Iris Diagnosis which is not strictly a part of TCM but is well worth learning for a broader approach to treatment. All of the areas of diagnosis on the body and ways of analyzing of the body can be used together to treat the body as a whole. The symptoms discovered are like red flags the patient is waving at you, begging you to see what his or her body is attempting to correct.

I will assume a standing knowledge of how to take a case history and what conclusions to draw and move on to a discussion of how you can detect chakra energy imbalance by using the tongue, pulse, abdomen, and tender chakra points with their reflexes on the limbs. The information gathered from the five areas of diagnosis and analysis mentioned below will give you the state and energetic condition of each major chakra.

TONGUE DIAGNOSIS

The tongue is an extremely useful tool not only in the traditional therapies but also in orthodox medicine. The tongue, as a whole, is said to be the outward expression of the inner economy, i.e., the stomach and intestines. When we have an upset stomach, the tongue exhibits altered coloring and texture. A clear tongue indicates strong vital force. When we change our diet or fast for any length of time, the tongue becomes furred, indicating the body's attempt to rid itself of toxins. Traditionally speaking, in order to detox the body we should fast as long as the tongue remains furred. As soon as the tongue clears, the fast should be halted. TCM practitioners know that tongue diagnosis measures much more than inner toxicity and infection. The tongue may be divided into areas that are associated with the internal organs. Figure 2.6 represents a typical diagram of a tongue with the internal organs shown in the traditional Five Elements' colors. There are many charts on tongue diagnosis. The illustration provided in this book represents a composite of a few different charts. The tongue may show the patterns of disease when analyzed, according to the Zang Fu system (or Eight Principles) of Heat and Cold, Emptiness and Fullness, Deficiency and Excess, and *Yin* and *Yang*. The corresponding archetypal changes in the tongue coating are redness (heat), yellow (interior), grey or black (cold and chronic), etc. Tongue diagnosis is a much-used and valued friend—a guide to ascertaining the root cause of a condition.

(See page 103, Figure 2.6. Traditional Tongue Diagnosis—TCM, and Figure 2.7. Traditional Tongue Diagnosis—Chakras.)

I have used this wonderful area of diagnosis to show you the energy states of the patient's major chakras. Chakra diagnosis using the tongue is a lot simpler than TCM tongue diagnosis: simply ascertain whether the corresponding area is *yin* or *yang*. *Yin* areas are thickly coated, dark, and grey or black. *Yang* areas are red, raw, or patchy. Figure 2.7 shows the correspondences of the chakras (and their colors). They are:

- The **Crown chakra** represents the "fire" organs of Heart and Pericardium systems and is located at the tip of the tongue. Redness and lack of coating at the tip represents heart and circulation imbalance plus a lack of grounding by the patient. They usually have hypertension and are in a great deal of stress and worry.

- The **Brow chakra** represents the "wood" organs of the Liver and Gall Bladder. The area is usually considered to be along the left side of the tongue but other charts place the two organs on both sides. A *yang* Brow chakra area represents inner anger and frustration or possible drug overdose—including many prescription drugs. I once had a patient with redness in this area who was mild and placid, but it was eventually discovered through liver function tests that he was suffering from long-term acetaminophen (paracetomol) poisoning. A *yin* Brow chakra region may indicate long-term liver poisoning or faulty diet (too much fatty food).

- The **Throat chakra** represents the "metal" Lung and Large Intestine organs. The Lungs are situated on the right hand side of the tongue, although some other charts might position this area just distal to the Pericardium. The Large Intestine is situated at the center of the tongue encompassing the Stomach region. This juxtaposition is common in reflected areas. The same thing occurs in Iris Diagnosis. On one hand, a *yang* Throat chakra region may indicate an acute infection either of the chest or bowel. On the other hand, a *yin* Throat chakra region may indicate a chronic lung or bowel condition. Alternatively, it may indicate suppression of thoughts, suppression of ideas, and inability to express oneself.

- The **Heart chakra** represents the "fire" Small Intestine and Triple Energizer organ system. The Heart chakra is situated between the tip and centre of the tongue. Not every tongue chart I have seen indicates the Triple Energizer. A *yang* Heart chakra region would indicate acute inflammation anywhere in the body, with enteritis being predominant. A *yin* Heart chakra region would indicate chronic bowel sluggishness, circulation imbalance such as varicose veins, and irregular body temperature (hypothalamus).

- The **Solar Plexus chakra** represents the "earth" organ of the Stomach. The position of the Solar Plexus chakra is at the center of the tongue. The tongue represents a reflected area of the body along with at least fourteen other areas. In each and every case the stomach and Solar Plexus chakra represent the earth and center of the reflected area, mimicking its position in the body. A *yang* Solar Plexus region represents gastritis, including acute allergic reactions. A *yin* Solar Plexus region means that there are long-term dietary problems, often of an allergic nature. The tongue often has a dirty yellow coating with chronic stomach energy imbalance.

- The **Sacral chakra** represents the "earth" organ of the Spleen. The position is between the center and the root of the tongue. A *yang* Sacral area indicates acute blood infection or gynecological condition. A *yin* Sacral region usually means chronic uterine congestion and conditions allied to the immune system.

• The **Base chakra** represents the "water" Kidney and Bladder organs. The Base chakra is situated at the very root of the tongue. It is difficult to ascertain a *yang* condition in this region due to its location but a *yin* condition where the darker coloring is more noticeable. With chronic spinal, kidney, and bladder conditions, the coloring is sometimes grey or black.

Traditional Pulse Diagnosis

There is little I say about this excellent form of analysis that has not been said a thousand times! Pulse diagnosis remains the crown jewel of TCM analysis. As TCM trained acupuncturists admit freely, pulse diagnosis is not easy to learn or to practice, but the rewards of being able to do it are infinite. In 1976 while earning my Licenciate in Acupuncture, I had the pleasure of attending a seminar in London given by a Chinese acupuncture professor named Doctor Lo who gave a talk on pulse diagnosis. At this stage my studies, *yin yang* terminology was a real headache to my Western medicine trained mind. When the theoretical side of his presentation was over, he asked for a volunteer to do some practical work with him. I volunteered, and he spent three to four minutes feeling my pulse and occasionally looking at my eyes and at my tongue. Then, he proceeded to tell me what problems I had at the time, what conditions I had suffered from over the previous twenty years, and—if I did not mend my ways—what I would suffer in the future. Everything he said was exactly correct. I was shocked. In hindsight, learning the power of pulse diagnosis first hand was the single most important incident in my training and convinced me that the study of Chinese medicine was worth doing and worth doing well.

The pulse diagnosis represents one of the oldest types of traditional diagnosis. Western trained practitioners are used to feeling for just *one* pulse at the distal end of the radial artery by the wrist. To be told that there are twelve interpretations of this one pulse can be a hard pill to swallow. Finding the different superficial and deep pulses is extremely demanding for the beginner who has not yet learned to feel even one pulse correctly. Furthermore, not only are there twelve pulses to learn, there are up to twenty-seven variations of each of the twelve pulses. The pulse may be superficial, floating, deep, slow, rapid, empty, full, slippery, choppy, thread-like, fine, weak, wiry, or one of many other variations. Figure 2.8 shows the positions of the twelve pulses that may be accessed by superficial and deep pressure on the radial artery as viewed by TCM. Figure 2.9 shows how the relative pulses may be interpreted to ascertain the state of the chakras at that moment in time. Both diagrams are color coded as before.

(See page 104, Figure 2.8. Traditional Pulse Diagnosis—TCM and Figure 2.9. Traditional Pulse Diagnosis—Chakras.)

The left wrist shows the energy quality of the Crown or Heart chakra, Brow chakra, and Base chakra, whereas the right wrist shows the energy quality of the Throat chakra, Solar Plexus or Sacral chakra, and Crown or Heart chakra. The energy quality of the Crown chakra may be determined at the left proximal superficial and the right distal deep positions. The energy quality of the Heart chakra is at the left proximal deep and right distal deep positions. The Solar Plexus chakra energy quality is ascertained at the right middle superficial position and the Sacral chakra at the right middle deep position. If this seems very complicated, the good news is that you do not need to ascertain and discern the many qualities of the pulse that have been described. You just need to get an overall sensation and feel of the pulse positions and how they differ from each other. You have to feel for obvious sluggishness (*yin*) or obvious hyperactivity (*yang*) to discern the chakra quality. This information is then added to what has been ascertained during the tongue diagnosis.

TRADITIONAL ABDOMINAL AND HARA DIAGNOSIS

The traditional Abdominal and *Hara* Diagnosis method of touch analysis forms part of TCM and Ayurvedic medicine although the latter system has a different abdominal reflex layout. Figure 2.10 shows a typical abdominal reflex areas diagram of the internal organs as used in TCM transposed with the associated chakras. Please note that the stomach

(Solar Plexus chakra) is once again in the centre of the area whereas the Crown and Base chakras are at the proximal and distal ends of the reflected area. This arrangement is common to all the reflected pathways and areas of the body.

(See page 105, Figure 2.10. Abdominal Diagnosis Areas—TCM Transposed to Chakras.)

Figure 2.11 shows *Hara* diagnosis regions that are typically used in *shiatsu*, yoga, reiki, and many other forms of healing. There is quite a substantial difference to the TCM abdominal reflex areas. I prefer *Hara* diagnosis because it seems to give a truer interpretation of what the patient's body is expressing. Figure 2.12 shows the *Hara* diagnosis regions transposed onto the chakra energy system. Please note that the same color coding applies as before.

(See pages 106 and 107, Figure 2.11. Traditional *Hara* Diagnosis—TCM and Figure 2.12. Traditional *Hara* Diagnosis—Chakras.)

Whichever concept you use, when you press the associated area with a gentle touch and elicit discomfort, this usually indicates an acute inflammatory *(yang)* state of the associated organ. Pain and discomfort discovered with a much deeper palpation indicates a more chronic and longstanding condition with the resultant deep energy changes *(yin)*. With a similarity to pulse diagnosis, when palpating the reflected chakra areas in the abdomen, often you will compare one side to the other, not necessarily feeling for whether one reflected area is *yin* or *yang*. Consequently, the whole abdominal region must be palpated before any conclusions may be drawn about energy imbalance and the possible treatment.

TENDER ACUPOINTS (MAJOR CHAKRAS)

It is a well known fact that when an acupoint needs treatment by acupuncture or acupressure there is a certain degree of tenderness at that acupoint. Tender points are a tried and tested method of analysis. A tender point is a signal that a particular acupoint is in a state of imbalance. It is also true that in addition to the acupoint requiring treatment being tender, the reflex of the point is also tender. Reflexes, reflected points, reflected areas, and pathways in the body have been my main study over the past thirty years. When imbalanced, each part of the body (organ, joint, muscle, etc.) reflects a need for treatment in one or more areas on the body. The major chakras are no exception to this rule. The main reflected points that are used in everyday practice are those on the feet and hands (see the chapter on Reflexology in *Healing with the Chakra Energy System* for additional information). Very little is known about the reflected points on the arms and legs. In a future book, *The Holistic Spine: Reflections and Associations,* I will outline that each vertebral level has a reflected point on the arms and legs as well as other regions of the body and that these may be used in both analysis and treatment. Reflected points are often more tender than the points that needs attention. They may be used in treatment, especially with acupressure and body reflexology, but I will describe them here in a purely analytical way. Figure 2.13 shows the anterior major chakras together with their relevant reflected points on the arm and leg.

(See page 108, Figure 2.13. Reflected Major Chakras on Arm and Leg.)

Please note that all the reflex points are *yin* points and are therefore situated on the anterior aspect of the arm or antro-medial aspect of the leg. When palpating these points, try not to be too enthusiastic—they will be tender to light touch. The discerning and experienced practitioner also recognizes different sensations when touching the point. If the reflected point is acutely sore, then the chakra is hyperactive and needs sedating. When the reflected point appears sluggish, then the chakra is sluggish and needs stimulating. Experience is the key: nothing happens overnight. Try this technique of testing and treating reflected points on as many patients as you can to learn the various meanings of the differences in feeling. The whole concept of tender reflected points in TCM makes for fascinating study—for many reasons I cannot logically see any difference between acupoints and reflex points. To me, each reflected point is an energetic extension of the central nervous system. Much of this work has been covered in my first two books on acupressure and reflextherapy, *Acupressure—Clinical Aspects in the Treatment of Musculo-Skeletal Conditions* and *Acupressure and Reflextherapy in Medical Conditions,* both published by Butterworth Heinemann. The various references and research into the reflected point's correlation with the central nervous system

(CNS) is covered in another book that is still in manuscript form called *Light Touch Reflextherapy.*

This concludes the part of the chapter dealing with analysis and diagnosis. It may, at first glance, seem to be a daunting task to transpose the TCM approach of the Five Elements, Pulse, Tongue, Abdominal, and *Hara* onto the chakra energy system. It takes time and patience. Once mastered, the feedback you get from your patients will make the extra time and effort worth your time.

ACUPUNCTURE POINTS USED WITH THE CHAKRA ENERGY SYSTEM

I will conclude this chapter with a list of the points that are required when using the chakra energy system with acupuncture. It describes the major chakra acupoints, minor chakra acupoints, and the Key points with instructions for needling procedures.

CROWN CHAKRA

- **Crown chakra point,** Gov 20—*Bai Hui,* is situated on the dorsal midline midway between the two auricular apices and only takes subcutaneous needling.
- **Key point (1),** TE 5—*Wai Guan,* is situated two cun proximal to the dorsal wrist crease between the ulna and radius: needle up to one inch perpendicular.
- **Key point (2),** Con 4—*Guanyuan,* is situated three cun below the umbilicus on the midline: needle one inch perpendicular.

BROW CHAKRA

- **Anterior Brow chakra point,** Extra (sometimes called Extra 3)—*Yintang,* is situated on the ventral midline between the eyebrows: needle subcutaneously.
- **Posterior Brow chakra point,** Gov 16—*Feng Fu,* is situated on the dorsal midline below the occipital protuberance: needle superficially.

- **Key point (1), SP 6**—*Sanyinjiao*, is situated three cun above the tip of the medial malleolus just posterior to the tibial border: needle one-half to one inch.
- **Key point (2), Gov 4**—*Mingmen*, is situated between the spinous processes of L2-L3 in the midline—needle one to on and one-half inches.

THROAT CHAKRA

- **Anterior Throat chakra point,** Con 22—*Tiantu*, is situated at the center of the suprasternal fossa one-half cun above the sternal notch: needle one-half inch.
- **Posterior Throat chakra point,** Gov 14—*Dazhui*, is situated between the seventh cervical and the spinous process of the first thoracic vertebra in the midline: needle one-half to one inch at a slight slant.
- **Key point (1), Con 6**—*Qihai*, is situated one and one-half cun below the umbilicus in the midline: needle one to two inches.
- **Key point (2), LR 5**—*Ligou*, is situated five cun superior to the medial malleolus on the posterior border of the tibia: needle one-half to one inch along posterior border of tibia.

HEART CHAKRA

- **Anterior Heart chakra point,** Con 17—*Shanzhong*, is situated in the center of the sternum half way between the nipples: needle superficially with needle pointed upwards.
- **Posterior Heart chakra point,** Gov 10—*Lingtai*, is situated below the spinous process of the sixth thoracic vertebra: needle one-half inch slightly upwards.
- **Key point (1), Gov 7**—*Zhongshu*, is situated below the spinous process of the tenth thoracic vertebra—needle one-half inch slightly upwards.

- **Key point (2)**, HT 1—*Jiquan,* is situated at the center of the axilla on the medial side of the auxiliary artery: needle one-half inch. Please note that some authorities consider this point to be forbidden to needle. Do not needle this point if you are unsure or have not been trained specifically to use this point.

SOLAR PLEXUS CHAKRA

- **Anterior Solar Plexus chakra point,** Con 14—*Jujue,* is situated six cun above the umbilicus in the midline: needle one inch obliquely downwards.
- **Posterior Solar Plexus chakra point,** Gov 6—*Jizhong,* is situated below the spinous process of the eleventh thoracic vertebra: needle one-half to one inch slightly upwards.
- **Key point (1)**, Con 17—*Shanzhong,* is situated in the center of the sternum half way between the nipples—needle superficially with needle pointed upwards.
- **Key point (2)**, TE 4—*Yangchi,* is situated in the depression of the posterior wrist crease—needle up to one-half inch perpendicular.

SACRAL CHAKRA

- **Anterior Sacral chakra point,** Con 6—*Qihai,* situated one and one-half cun below the umbilicus: needle one to two inches perpendicular.
- **Posterior Sacral chakra point,** Gov 3—*Yaoyangguan,* is situated in the interspace between L4 and L5: needle one inch with needle inclined upwards.
- **Key point (1)**, Gov 12—*Shenzu,* situated below the spinous process of the third thoracic vertebra: needle one-half inch slightly upwards.
- **Key point (2)**, PC 3—*Quze,* situated in the center of the transverse cubical crease at the ulnar side of the biceps tendon: needle one-half inch perpendicular.

BASE CHAKRA

- **Anterior Base chakra point,** Con 2—*Qugu,* is situated at the superior border of the pubic symphysis on the midline: needle one to one and one-half inches perpendicular.

- **Poster Base chakra point,** Gov 2—*Yaoshu,* is situated at the junction between the coccyx and sacrum: needle one-half inch obliquely upwards.

- **Key point (1),** Con 22—*Tiantu,* is situated at the center of the suprasternal fossa one-half cun above the sternal notch: needle one-half inch.

- **Key point (2),** LR 8—*Ququan,* is situated at the medial end of the transverse crease of the knee joint in a depression at the anterior border of the semi-membranous tendon: needle one inch perpendicular.

SPLEEN CHAKRA

- **Spleen chakra point,** SP 16(L)—*Fuai,* is situated seven cun directly below the nipple lateral to Con 11: needle perpendicular to eight-tenths of an inch.

- **Key point,** Gov 8—*Jinsuo,* is situated directly below the spinous process of the ninth thoracic vertebra: needle one-half inch slightly upwards.

FOOT CHAKRA

- **Foot chakra point,** KID 1—*Yongquan,* is situated in the depression at the junction of the anterior and middle third of the sole in a depression between the second and third metatarsophalangeal joint when the toes are flexed: needle up to one-half inch.

- **Key point,** HT 6—*Yinxi,* is situated on the ulnar side of the wrist, on the radial side of the flexor carpi ulnaris, one-half cun superior to HT 7: needle one-third inch perpendicular.

HAND CHAKRA

- **Hand chakra point,** PC 8—*Laogong,* is situated in the center of the palm between the middle and ring fingers, adjacent to the third metacarpal bone: needle perpendicular approximately one-third of an inch.
- **Key point,** KID 3—*Taixi,* is situated midway between the tip of the medial malleolus and the Achilles tendon: needle up to one-half inch toward the Achilles tendon.

KNEE CHAKRA

- **Knee chakra point,** BL 40—*Weizhong,* is situated in the exact midpoint of the popliteal fossa: needle approximately one inch perpendicular.
- **Key point,** SI 7—*Zhizheng,* is situated three cun proximal to the wrist on the ulnar border of the forearm: needle one-half inch perpendicular.

ELBOW CHAKRA

- **Elbow chakra point,** PC 3—*Quze,* is situated in the center of the transverse cubical crease at the ulnar side of the biceps brachii: needle one-half to one inch perpendicular.
- **Key point,** BL 59—*Fuyang,* is situated three cun superior to BL 60 posterior to the external malleolus: needle up to one inch perpendicular.

GROIN CHAKRA

- **Groin chakra point,** ST 30—*Qichong,* is situated five cun inferior to the umbilicus two cun lateral to the midline: needle one inch perpendicular.
- **Key point,** PC 7—*Daling,* is situated at the center of the transverse wrist crease between palmaris longus and flexor carpi radialis tendons: needle up to one-half inch perpendicular.

CLAVICULAR CHAKRA

- **Clavicular chakra point,** KID 27—*Shufu,* is situated in the depression between the first rib and the lower border of the clavicle two cun lateral to the mid-line: needle one-half inch obliquely.
- **Key point,** LR 8—*Ququan,* is situated at the medial end of the transverse crease of the knee joint—needle one to one and one-half inches perpendicular.

SHOULDER CHAKRA

- **Shoulder chakra point,** LI 15—*Jianyu,* is situated at the anterior and inferior border of the acromioclavicular joint inferior to the acromion when the arm is in abduction: needle one inch obliquely downwards when arm is in adduction.
- **Key point,** ST 40—*Fenglong,* situated eight cun below the knee one-half cun lateral to ST 38: needle one to one and one-half inches perpendicular.

NAVEL CHAKRA

- **Navel chakra point,** KID 16—*Huangshu,* situated one-half cun lateral to the umbilicus: needle up to one inch perpendicular.
- **Key point,** LI 15—*Quchi,* is situated in the depression at the lateral end of the transverse cubical crease when elbow is half-flexed: needle up to one and one-half inches perpendicular.

INTERCOSTAL CHAKRA

- **Intercostal chakra point,** SP 21—*Dabao,* is situated on the mid-auxiliary line in the sixth intercostal space—needle one-half inch obliquely.
- **Key point,** GB 37—*Guangming,* is situated five cun above the tip of the lateral malleolus close to the anterior border of the fibula: needle one inch perpendicular.

EAR CHAKRA

- **Ear chakra point,** TE 17—*Yifeng,* is situated posterior to the ear lobe in a depression between the angle of the mandible and the mastoid process: needle one-half inch perpendicular or one inch obliquely forward and upward.

- **Key point,** TE 4—*Yangchi,* is situated in the depression of the transverse wrist crease of the dorsum of the wrist between the tendon extensions of the extensor digitorum: needle up to one-half inch perpendicular.

TREATMENT OF PAIN

I should imagine that well over ninety percent of our time is spent in treating pain. There are many excellent acupuncture techniques for treating pain and several specific acupoints that historically have been found to be the most useful in pain relief. What I am presenting to you is a different approach to pain relief—an approach using the minor chakras. I mention specific conditions in detail in Chapter Four. In this Chapter I offer you an alternative to the usual acupuncture methods that may appear so controversial it would be heresy to some practitioners. Chapter Three is based on my pioneering work over twenty-five years of using these methods clinically. It does *not* present an evidence-based methodology. I present here my original work—not yet subject to scientific scrutiny. Chakra acupuncture, and in particular pain relief using the minor chakras, represents an excellent topic for a research project. I would welcome someone to do a scientific study and would assist in any way that I could.

ACUPUNCTURE TREATMENT OF PAIN

The following are the most commonly used methods of acupuncture to treat pain:

- The use of local points over or around the pain site either by ordinary or periosteal needling and done manually or using electroacupuncture.
- The use of local points as above with the addition of a distal point (or points) to enhance the treatment. The distal points may be along the same meridian or one of the classical Great points used

in pain relief, e.g., LI 4, SP 6, etc. Treatment can be performed manually or with electroacupuncture.

- The use of trigger points or myofascial points that historically have been proven useful in ameliorating pain. The concept of modern Western (not TCM) acupuncture has centered on the use of trigger points.
- As well as stainless steel needle acupuncture such modalities as copper and zinc needles, biomagnets, TENS, lasers, and acupressure may all be performed as well as several types of electro-acupuncture.

If there are so many types of pain relief acupuncture that have been scientifically proved to work, what is the point in creating another one? Many methods of pain relief employ techniques that I sarcastically call "symptomatic pin-pricking." In other words, "If it hurts, stick a needle in it!" The reason why these methods have taken off in the West is that often they work. Western acupuncture generally does not treat the *cause* of the pain but rather eases it or enables the body to suppress it. In over thirty years of practicing acupuncture I have heard both sides of the argument about Western versus Traditional and symptomatic relief versus treating the cause. I am utterly convinced that by just treating the pain syndrome and ignoring the underlying cause (which may be some considerable distance from the pain site), a great injustice is being done to the patient. We need to have a system of acupuncture that combines the pain relief quality with treating the cause. I believe pain relief and treatment of the source of the pain can be achieved by using the method of treating the minor chakras that I discovered. The influence of the minor chakras does not reach a spiritual level the way the major chakras do, but their influence reaches the emotional body, which is the subtle body that is often the area of etiology in pain syndromes. Pain anywhere in the physical body, apart from obvious traumatic, injurious, and post-surgical etiology often falls under the domain of emotional imbalance. Having stated that, the minor chakras will ease pain caused by injury as well as emotional pain. In fact, the unbelievable thing about using these chakra points in pain relief is that the cause of the discomfort is immaterial. I have stated this fact on numerous occasions in workshops, in seminars, in lectures, and in print. I say it with the utmost conviction with my practical experience in evidence.

USE OF THE MINOR CHAKRAS IN PAIN RELIEF

The only minor chakra that is not discussed in this chapter is the Spleen chakra which is used more in combination treatment with the Solar Plexus and Sacral chakras in chronic conditions than alone. Therefore the Spleen chakra will be fully discussed in Chapter Four. The other twenty minor chakras are to be found on the periphery of the body. As discussed in Chapter One, the peripheral twenty minor chakras (ten bilaterally) are reflected (reflex) points of the major chakras as well as being powerful acupoints in their own right. In the early 1980s, I discovered accidentally when minor chakra points were used in acupuncture on patients, they were experiencing analgesia in areas of the body that were sometimes quite remote to where the needles had been inserted. This discovery heralded a period of feverish activity on my part. Prior to using the minor chakras as treatment entities in their own right, they had only been used in combination treatment with the major chakras or as individual acupoints for other procedures. It took several months of painstaking research to discover the minor chakra Key points, associated meridians, and areas of the body affected by them. The minor chakras may be used for treating both acute and chronic pain, but their great asset is in the treatment of long standing (sometimes intransigent) pain.

For the purposes of these procedures, the body is divided up into five different areas that are associated with a set of coupled minor chakras—each called a Schedule. For using each Schedule you need to know the following:

• The acupoint of the minor chakra
• The acupoint of its Key point
• The acupoint of the coupled minor chakra
• The acupoint of its Key point

The Schedules 1-5 are as follows:

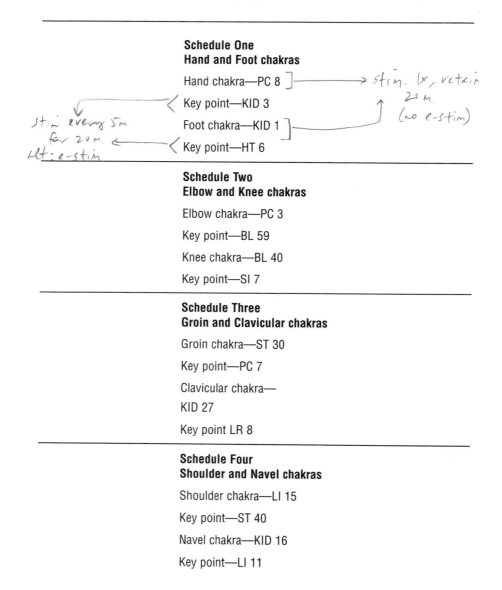

Schedule One
Hand and Foot chakras

Hand chakra—PC 8   *stim. 1x, retain 20 m. (no e-stim)*

Key point—KID 3

Foot chakra—KID 1

Key point—HT 6

stim every 5m for 20 m. Lt: e-stim

Schedule Two
Elbow and Knee chakras

Elbow chakra—PC 3

Key point—BL 59

Knee chakra—BL 40

Key point—SI 7

Schedule Three
Groin and Clavicular chakras

Groin chakra—ST 30

Key point—PC 7

Clavicular chakra—

KID 27

Key point LR 8

Schedule Four
Shoulder and Navel chakras

Shoulder chakra—LI 15

Key point—ST 40

Navel chakra—KID 16

Key point—LI 11

Schedule Five
Ear and Intercostal chakras

Ear chakra—TE 17

Key point—TE 4

Intercostal chakra—SP 21

Key point—GB 37

Schedule One

PAIN AREAS TREATED

- Anterior head and scalp above the eyes
- Posterior head and scalp to include the cervical spine to C7
- Hands and wrists
- Feet and ankle

PAIN CONDITIONS TREATED

- Metatarsalgia
- Foot pain
- Hand and wrist pain
- Headaches of any type
- Head shingles (herpes zoster) pain
- Cervical pain due to osteoarthritic changes
- Sensory and motor pain of all the preceding

(See page 109, Figure 3.1. Minor Chakras Pain Relief—Schedule One.)

Schedule Two

PAIN AREAS TREATED

- Mid-forearm to mid-arm—front, and back
- Mid-thigh to mid-calf—front and back
- Lumbar spine, sacral region, and pelvis

PAIN CONDITIONS TREATED

- Chronic and acute elbow and knee pain, including arthritis
- Tennis elbow
- Golfers elbow
- Medial and lateral ligament pain
- Lower back pain
- Lumbosacral arthritis pain
- Sacroiliac pain

(See page 110, Figure 3.2. Minor Chakras Pain Relief—Schedule Two.)

Schedule Three

PAIN AREAS TREATED

- Clavicles
- Throat
- Scapula
- Chest front and back, except thoracic spine
- Groin
- Adductor muscles
- Thigh down to mid-thigh—front and back

PAIN CONDITIONS TREATED

- All painful chronic and acute respiratory conditions
- Cardiovascular pain
- Angina

- Groin pain
- Uterine and testicular discomfort
- Cystitis

(See page 111, Figure 3.3. Minor Chakras Pain Relief—Schedule Three.)

SCHEDULE FOUR

PAIN AREAS TREATED

- Shoulders—front and back
- Stomach and abdomen
- Sinuses
- Nose
- Mouth and teeth
- Chin
- Neck above throat

PAIN CONDITIONS TREATED

- Shoulder joint—capsule and girdle
- Conditions including the pain of frozen shoulder
- Painful stomach and abdominal conditions
- Sinusitis
- Catarrhal pain
- Toothache

(See page 112, Figure 3.4. Minor Chakra Pain Relief—Schedule Four.)

SCHEDULE FIVE

PAIN AREAS TREATED

- Eyes
- Ears
- Temporomandibular joint region

- Thoracic spine, ribs seven through twelve
- Posterior and lateral aspect of trunk (loin)

PAIN CONDITIONS TREATED

- Facial shingles
- Intercostal shingles
- Eye strain
- Earache
- Sinusitis
- Temporomandibular joint disorder (TMJ) pain
- Painful kidney conditions

(See page 113, Figure 3.5. Minor Chakras Pain Relief—Schedule Five.)

Figure 3.6 shows a composite picture of the pain relief areas together with the minor chakra points and Key points.

(See page 114, Figure 3.6. Pain Relief Areas.)

TECHNIQUE

- First you need to ascertain where the pain is—this could be muscular, joint, sensory, sympathetic, or spinal referred pain that affects the dermatome or nerve.

  When you have decided on the area of pain to be treated, both Key points are needled and stimulated for a few seconds. It is very important that the Key points are stimulated for a few seconds every five minutes for the twenty minutes that they are in situ. It is imperative that the patient experiences the de qui sensation, so you know that the needles are in the correct position.

- Once the Key points have been stimulated for the first time, needle both minor chakra points. Stimulate the needle just enough to experience *de qui* but no longer than that. The minor chakra needles remain still for the remainder of the treatment time of approximately twenty minutes.

- When an overlap of the pain area Schedules occurs (very common), the second Schedule may be treated at the same time so that there will be a total of eight needles *in situ* at the same time. Do not attempt to treat more than two Schedules at the same time. With complex cases exhibiting more than two pain areas, start with the one that has the most acute presenting symptoms.

- Electroacupuncture may be used to keep the Key points stimulated but on no account should it be used with the minor chakra points.

- Pain relief chakra acupuncture using the minor chakras may be used in isolation in any one treatment session or in combination with other chakra acupuncture techniques.

ASSOCIATED MERIDIANS

Each Schedule has two meridians with which it is associated. If, for any reason, the desired results are not being achieved the associated meridians may be used as a back-up system. The meridians may be stroked with the palms in the direction of energy flow, be stimulated with a plum blossom hammer, or be needled at its Source point. The following table and the previous illustrations provide the associated meridians to each schedule and source point:

Schedule	Meridians	Source Points
One	Heart	HT 7
	Kidney	KID 3 (same as Key point)
Two	Small Intestine	SI 4
	Bladder	BL 64
Three	Liver	LR 3
	Pericardium	PC 7 (same as Key point)
Four	Large Intestine	LI 4
	Stomach	ST 42
Five	Triple Energizer	TE 4 (same as Key point)
	Gall Bladder	GB 40

Only use the associated meridians when the patient expresses no appreciable pain relief after approximately fifteen minutes following needling. You have a choice of stimulating the Source point (either manually or with electroacupuncture) or stroking the meridian with the palm of the hand.

CONCLUSION

I have invented a new approach to the treatment of pain by using the minor chakras with acupuncture. You might be reading this short chapter with incredulity, because it is very different to the usual approach to pain relief. I can assure you that I have taught this method for the past two decades and have witnessed the doubt and disbelief on the faces of my delegates turn to wonder and amazement when they realize that it works! I urge you to try it and witness the results for yourself. You will not be disappointed.

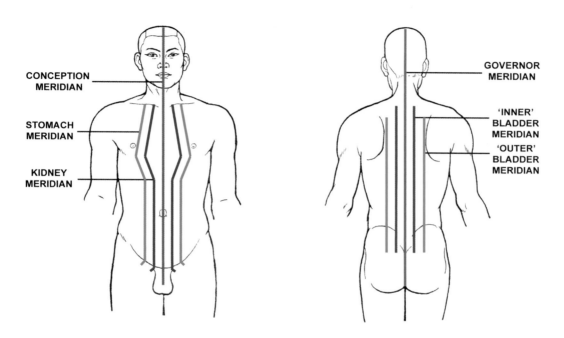

FIGURE 2.1. *Diagrammatic Representation of the Conception, Governor, Stomach, Kidney, and Bladder Meridians*

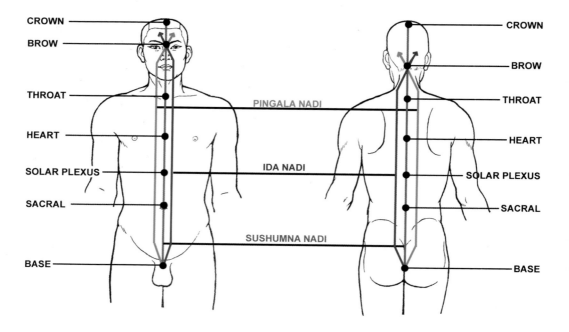

FIGURE 2.2. *Representation of the Sushumna, Ida, and Pingala Nadis (One)*

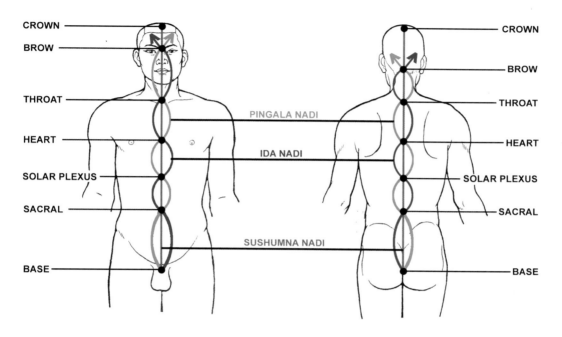

FIGURE 2.3. *Representation of the Sushumna, Ida, and Pingala Nadis (Two)*

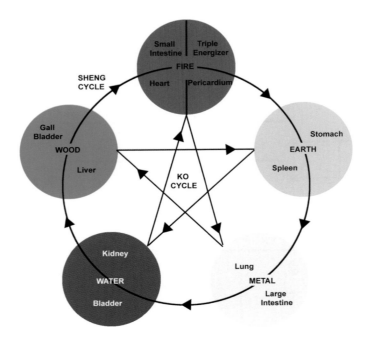

FIGURE 2.4. *Law of Five Elements—TCM*

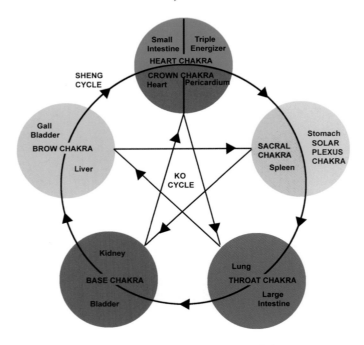

FIGURE 2.5. *Law of Five Elements—Chakras*

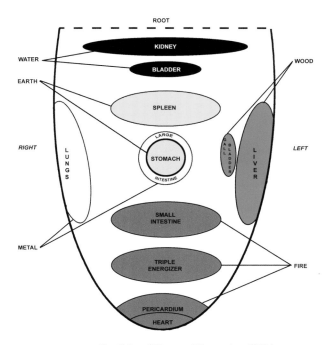

FIGURE 2.6. *Traditional Tongue Diagnosis—TCM*

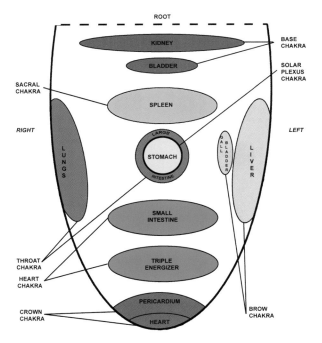

FIGURE 2.7. *Traditional Tongue Diagnosis—Chakras*

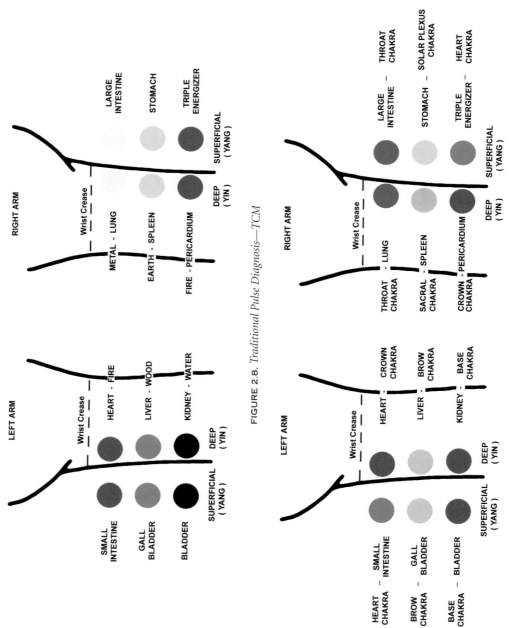

FIGURE 2.8. *Traditional Pulse Diagnosis—TCM*

FIGURE 2.9. *Traditional Pulse Diagnosis—Chakras*

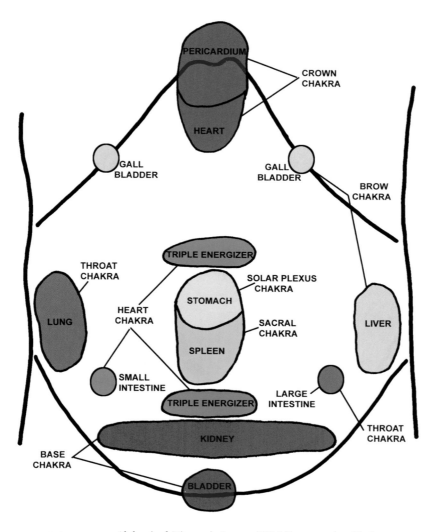

FIGURE 2.10. *Abdominal Diagnosis Areas—TCM Transposed to Chakras*

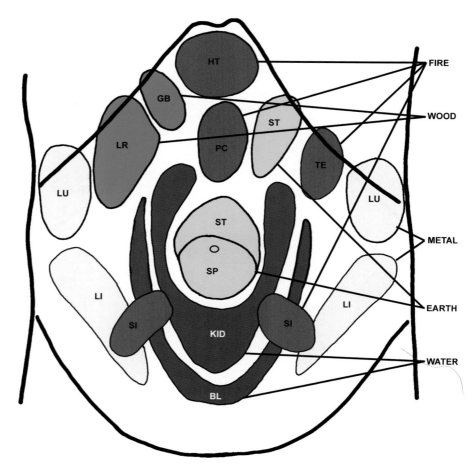

PC	PERICARDIUM	KID	KIDNEY
HT	HEART	BL	BLADDER
SI	SMALL INTESTINE	ST	STOMACH
TE	TRIPLE ENERGIZER	SP	SPLEEN
LU	LUNG	LR	LIVER
LI	LARGE INTESTINE	GB	GALLBLADDER

FIGURE 2.11. *Traditional Hara Diagnosis—TCM*

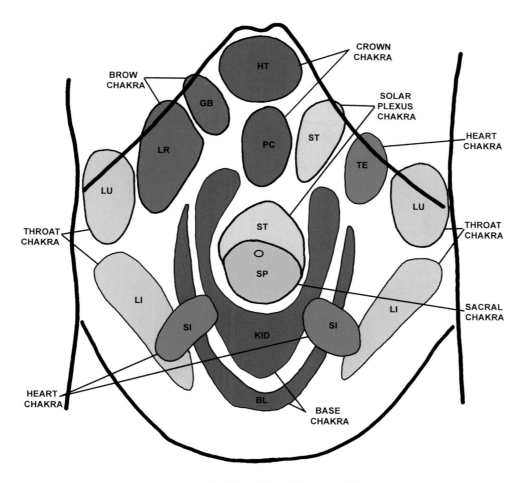

FIGURE 2.12. *Traditional Hara Diagnosis—Chakras*

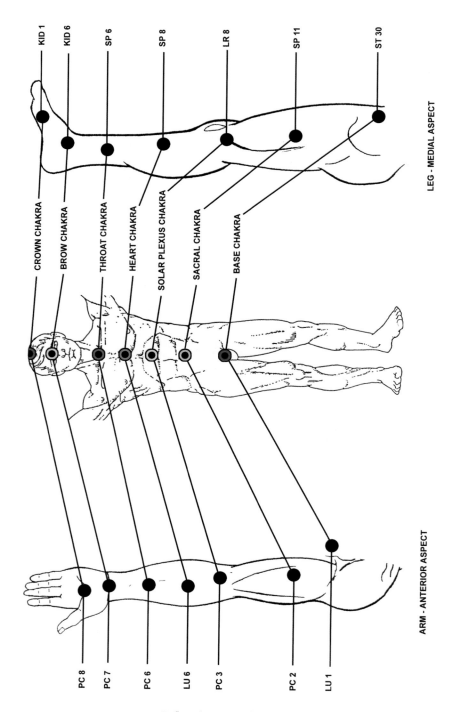

FIGURE 2.13. *Reflected Major Chakras on Arm and Leg*

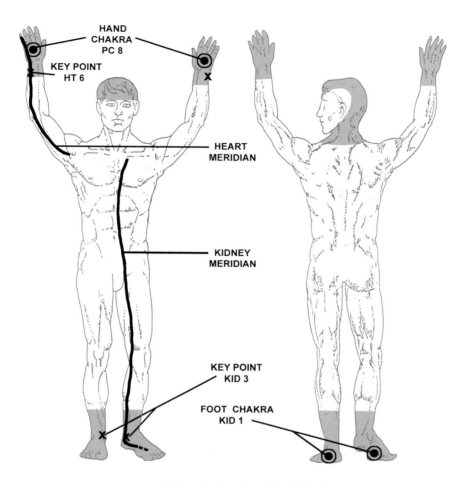

FIGURE 3.1. *Minor Chakras Pain Relief—Schedule One*

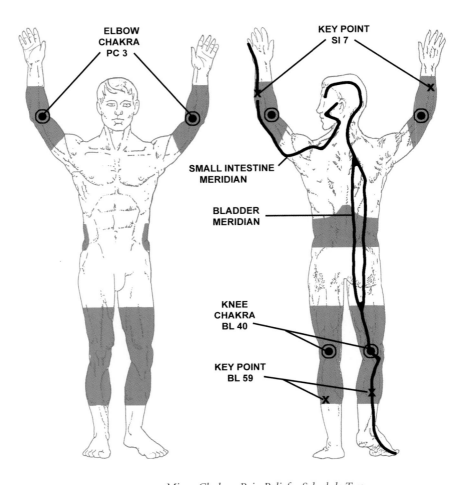

FIGURE 3.2. *Minor Chakras Pain Relief—Schedule Two*

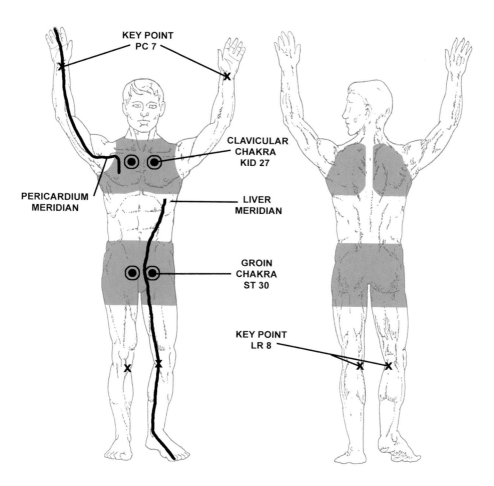

FIGURE 3.3. *Minor Chakras Pain Relief—Schedule Three*

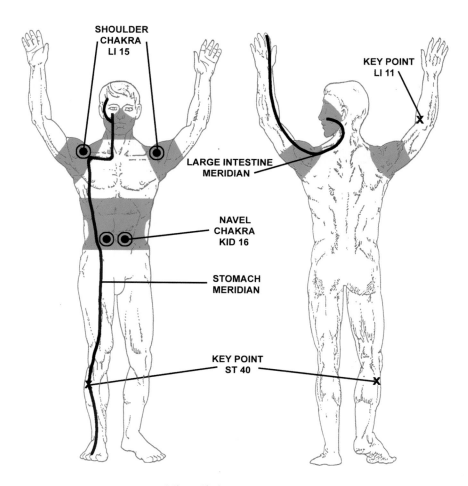

FIGURE 3.4. *Minor Chakra Pain Relief—Schedule Four*

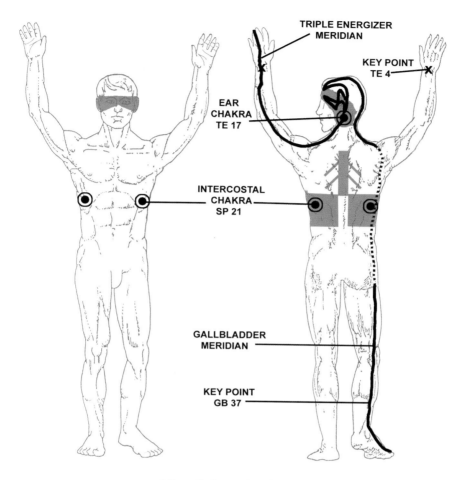

FIGURE 3.5. *Minor Chakras Pain Relief—Schedule Five*

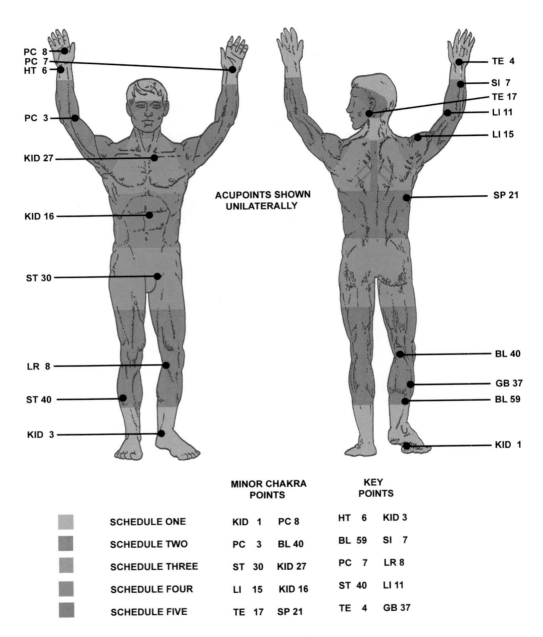

**ACUPOINTS SHOWN
UNILATERALLY**

	MINOR CHAKRA POINTS		KEY POINTS	
SCHEDULE ONE	KID 1	PC 8	HT 6	KID 3
SCHEDULE TWO	PC 3	BL 40	BL 59	SI 7
SCHEDULE THREE	ST 30	KID 27	PC 7	LR 8
SCHEDULE FOUR	LI 15	KID 16	ST 40	LI 11
SCHEDULE FIVE	TE 17	SP 21	TE 4	GB 37

FIGURE 3.6. *Pain Relief Areas*

CHAPTER FOUR

TREATMENT OF CHRONIC CONDITIONS

ACUPUNCTURE TREATMENT OF INDIVIDUAL CHAKRAS

Once it has been ascertained which chakra requires treatment, there are several ways in which one can proceed to treat the energy imbalanced chakra using acupuncture. Firstly it is imperative that the treated chakra is the correct one and, when treating multiple chakras, that the treatment of the chakras is carried out in a sequential order. The order of treatment is based on the general symptomatology that is presented at consultation. As stated before, more than one chakra may be treated (not at the same time unless it is a combination of major and minor), but they must be treated in order of priority. Symptoms may be gauged as being purely local and topical to being very broad and systemic. It does not matter when using chakra acupuncture, because the cause of the condition or disease *(dis-ease)* is addressed each and every time. Therefore mild mental, emotional, hormonal, organic, endocrine, and musculo-skeletal conditions may all be treated with these methods. Depending on the symptomatology, the following may be employed:

- Balancing and treatment of the affected major chakras only
- Combination treatment of major and minor chakras in chronic and complex cases
- Balancing and treating the minor chakras in pain relief (see Chapter Three)

- Hormonal production using the major chakras, the eight extraordinary meridians, and Bladder 1

BALANCING AND TREATMENT OF THE MAJOR CHAKRAS ONLY

The following major chakra treatments give the acupoints to be needled and the order that should be carried out in the treatment. Please note that both of the peripheral Key points have to be used in acupuncture whereas just one needs to be used (if at all) in acupressure. Where it states that either the anterior or posterior aspect of the major chakra is needled, both may be treated if desired. Placing the patient on his or her side will accommodate this. Posterior major chakra points are usually reserved for acute and musculo-skeletal conditions and the anterior aspect with chronic, organic, and emotional imbalance. The following listings show typical symptoms for each major chakra imbalance and are not exhaustive. The number of treatment sessions required depends on the chronicity of the problem—the usual rules of acupuncture apply here. What you will find, however, is that you will require far fewer treatments to achieve your goal than with standard TCM.

CROWN CHAKRA

TYPICAL SYMPTOMATOLOGY

Symptoms of the Crown chakra include vertigo, hypertension, right-sided migraine, symptoms associated with some upper motor neural conditions, e.g., multiple sclerosis (MS), right eye symptoms, brittle nails, lackluster hair, melancholia, depression, and delusion.

ACUPUNCTURE TREATMENT

1. Stimulate the Key points—Con 4 and TE 5. Sedate the chakra point—Con 20.
2. Sedate the coupled major chakra (Base) at either Con 2 or Gov 2.
3. Reinforce the treatment by stimulating the Source point of the associated meridian—Triple Energizer—TE 4.

Brow chakra

TYPICAL SYMPTOMATOLOGY

Symptoms of the Brow chakra include headache, migraine, chronic catarrh, infectious and contagious disease, left eye symptoms, deafness and altered hearing, arthritis of the cervical spine, cranial base conditions, vertebral artery conditions, stress-related symptoms, anxiety-related symptoms, anger, rage, Ménière's disease, adverse energy syndromes (e.g., headache reaction to microwave, photocopiers, and color television), and catarrh.

ACUPUNCTURE TREATMENT

1. Stimulate the Key points—Gov 4 and SP 6.
2. Sedate the chakra point—either (or both) Gov 16 or Extra 1 (*Yintang*).
3. Sedate the coupled major (Base) at either Gov 2 or Con 2.
4. Reinforce the treatment by stimulating the Source point of the associated meridian—Gall Bladder—GB 40.

Throat Chakra

TYPICAL SYMPTOMATOLOGY

Symptoms of the Throat Chakra include migraine, acute and chronic sore throats, tonsillitis, asthma, bronchitis, and other acute or chronic respiratory conditions, loss of taste, colitis, irritable bowel syndrome, ileocecal valve syndromes, constipation, diarrhea, cervicothoracic symptoms, shyness, and introverted behavior.

ACUPUNCTURE TREATMENT

1. Stimulate the Key points—Con 6 and LR 5.
2. Sedate the chakra point—either or both Gov 14 or Con 22.
3. Sedate the coupled major chakra (Sacral) at Gov 3 or Con 6.
4. Reinforce the treatment by stimulating the Source point of the associated meridians—Large Intestine and Lung—LI 4 and LU 9.

HEART CHAKRA

TYPICAL SYMPTOMATOLOGY

Heart chakra conditions include tachycardia, angina, post-surgical cardiac trauma, poor circulation (cold hands and feet), varicosities, nausea, vertigo, mid-thoracic pain, mild scoliosis, anxiety, tearfulness, and sequential nervous breakdown.

ACUPUNCTURE TREATMENT

1. Stimulate the Key points—Gov 7 and HT 1.
2. Sedate the chakra points—either or both Gov 10 or Con 17.
3. Sedate the couple major chakra (Solar Plexus)—Gov 6 or Con 12.
4. Reinforce the treatment by stimulating the Source point of the associated meridians—Heart and Small Intestine—HT 7 and SI 4.

SOLAR PLEXUS CHAKRA

TYPICAL SYMPTOMATOLOGY

Solar Plexus Chakra symptoms include stomach conditions, ulcers, gall bladder colic, glandular fever, chronic fatigue syndrome or myalgic encephalomyelitis (ME), skin conditions (such as eczema and acne), allergies of all kinds—including hay fever, lower thoracic spinal conditions, upper lumbar spinal conditions, anxiety, and depression. Please note that Solar Plexus chakra imbalance may also give rise to cancerous growths, diabetes, and hepatitis. By law, no non-registered medical practitioner may state that he or she is treating these conditions. However, it is perfectly permissible to treat patients who have these conditions, so long as practitioners make it clear that no cure is sought. Chakra acupuncture is wonderful for treating the *person* who has these conditions.

ACUPUNCTURE TREATMENT

1. Stimulate the Key points—Con17 and TE 4.
2. Sedate the chakra point—either or both Gov 6 or Con 12.
3. Sedate the coupled major chakra—Heart—at Gov 10 or Con 17.

4. Reinforce the treatment by stimulating the Source point of the associated meridians—Liver and Stomach—LR 3 and ST 42.

SACRAL CHAKRA

TYPICAL SYMPTOMATOLOGY

Symptoms of the Sacral Chakra include intestinal conditions, fatigue, low vitality, chronic sore throats, impotence, low or high libido, menstrual irregularities, menopausal symptoms, edema, swollen ankles, some rheumatoid factor conditions, lumbar pain, arthritis, and depression.

ACUPUNCTURE TREATMENT

1. Stimulate the Key points—Gov 12 and PC 3.
2. Sedate the chakra points—either or both Gov 3 or Con 6.
3. Sedate the coupled chakra—Throat at Gov 14 or Con 22.
4. Reinforce the treatment by stimulating the Source point of the associated meridians—Spleen and Pericardium—SP 3 and PC 7.

BASE CHAKRA

TYPICAL SYMPTOMATOLOGY

Base chakra symptoms include osteoarthritis, ankylosing spondylitis, some rheumatoid factor conditions, lumbosacral arthritis, lumbosacral pain, chronic tiredness, lethargy, stiff joints, nephritis, acute cystitis, chronic cystitis, gravitational ulcers, various bone diseases—particularly Scheuermann's disease, depression, and low spirits.

ACUPUNCTURE TREATMENT

1. Stimulate the Key points—Con 22 and LR 8.
2. Sedate the chakra points—either or both Gov 2 or Con 2.
3. Sedate the coupled major chakra—either Crown or Brow at Gov 20 or Extra 1 (Yintang).
4. Reinforce the treatment by stimulating the Source point of the associated meridians—Kidney and Bladder—KID 3 and BL 64.

The standard rules of acupuncture apply when giving treatment using the major chakras. Allow approximately twenty minutes for each set of points before moving to another formula.

COMBINATION OF MAJOR AND MINOR CHAKRAS IN CHRONIC AND COMPLEX CONDITIONS

When you treat a patient's condition and its affected chakra according to his or her symptoms without a positive response, it may be necessary to use a combination of major and minor chakras. The combination approach works very well in long standing and complex cases. The various associations are listed in Chapter One. For easy reference, they are as follows:

- The **Crown** chakra is coupled with the **Hand** and **Foot** minor chakras.
- The **Brow** chakra is coupled with the **Groin** and **Clavicular** minor chakras.
- The **Throat** chakra is coupled with the **Shoulder** and **Navel** minor chakras.
- The **Heart** chakra is coupled with the **Ear** and **Intercostal** minor chakras.
- The **Solar Plexus** is coupled with the **Sacral** major and the **Spleen** minor chakras.
- The **Sacral** chakra is coupled with the **Solar Plexus** major and the **Spleen** minor chakra.
- The **Base** chakra is coupled with the **Knee** and **Elbow** minor chakras.

The above six combinations incorporate the seven major and all twenty-one minor chakras. Please note that the Spleen chakra, although given minor chakra status, is very much the odd one out regarding positioning, symptomatology, and function. It is often said that the Spleen represents the eighth major chakra. The remaining twenty chakras are all peripheral points and are bilateral (see Chapter Three for full information on the minor chakras). Please note that the Crown, Brow, Throat, Heart, and Base

major chakras are each coupled with two of the peripheral minor chakras
(which are, in turn, coupled with each other) and that the Solar Plexus,
Sacral, and Spleen chakras make an extremely powerful combination.
Thus, the whole system of the physical, emotional, and mental make-up of
a person can be assessed and treated using one of the six chakra combinations. Also, each of the six combinations has two associated meridians
which may be used to supplement any treatment. The two meridians are
comprised of one *yang* and one *yin* meridian, thus adding to the holistic
approach. The following table denotes the acupoints required for each
treatment.

Combination Chakra	Yin Meridian	Yang Meridian	Key Points	Chakra Points	Meridian Source Points
Crown **Hand** **Foot**	Heart	Gall Bladder	Con 4 TE 5 KID 3 HT 6	Gov 20 PC 8 KID 1	HT 7 GB 40
Brow **Groin** **Clavicular**	Pericardium	Stomach	Gov 4 SP 6 PC 7 LR 8	Yintang ST 30 KID 27	PC 7 ST 42
Throat **Shoulder** **Navel**	Lung	Large Intestine	Con 6 LR 5 ST 40 LI 11	Con 22 LI 15 KID 16	LU 9 LI 4
Heart **Ear** **Intercostal**	Spleen	Triple Energizer	Gov 7 HT 1 TE 4 GB 37	Con 17 TE 17 SP 21	SP 3 TE 4
Solar Plexus **Sacral** **Spleen**	Liver	Small Intestine	TE 4 Gov 12 PC3 Gov 8 Con 17	Con 14 Con 6 SP 16	LR 3 SI 4
Base **Elbow** **Knee**	Kidney	Bladder	Con 22 LR 8 BL59 SI 7	Con 2 PC 3 BL 40	KID 3 BL 64

SYMPTOMATOLOGY OF THE COMBINED CHAKRAS

The following represents only a few named conditions that are treatable with combination chakra acupuncture—there are many more.

CROWN, HAND, AND FOOT

The combination of Crown, Head, and Foot chakras can treat head shingles (herpes zoster), cervical spondylosis, metatarsalgia—and other chronic foot maladies, vertigo, hypertension, headaches, migraines, upper motor neuron imbalance (not as a cure but to ease symptoms), and anxiety.

BROW, GROIN, AND CLAVICULAR

The combination of Brow, Groin, and Clavicular chakras treats migraines, cervical spondylosis, catarrh sinusitis, chronic sinusitis, adverse energy reactions, infections, infectious diseases, altered hearing, dizziness, some chronic respiratory conditions, and some chronic genitourinary conditions.

THROAT, SHOULDER, AND NAVEL

The combination of Throat, Shoulder, and Naval chakras treats asthma, chronic respiratory conditions, chronic sore throats, tonsillitis, thoracic outlet syndrome, colitis, irritable bowel syndrome, diverticulitis, frozen shoulder of non-traumatic etiology, anxiety, paranoia, and introversion.

HEART, EAR, AND INTERCOSTAL

The combination of Heart, Ear, and Intercostal chakras treats thoracic shingles (herpes zoster), some facial neuralgia, mid-thoracic scoliosis, general chronic cardiac conditions, circulation conditions, palpitation, tachycardia, varicosities, benign cysts, and growths.

SOLAR PLEXUS, SACRAL, AND SPLEEN

The combination of Solar Plexus, Sacral, and Spleen chakras treats conditions of the auto-immune system, glandular fever, chronic fatigue syndrome—also known as myalgic encephalomyelitis (ME), malignancies (not as a cure and in conjunction with other therapies), eczema, hay fever, various allergies, fatigue, lymphatic obstructions, edema, menopausal imbalance, menstrual imbalance, impotence (in conjunction with other therapies), rheumatoid arthritis, anxiety, and depression.

BASE, ELBOW, AND KNEE

The combination of Base, Elbow, and Knee chakras treats chronic spinal conditions, ankylosing spondylitis, lumbosacral arthritis, arthritic changes of the elbow and knee, general joint stiffness, chronic cystitis, nephritis, bone-related conditions, fatigue, severe depression, delusions, and inability to center.

ORDER OF TREATMENT

When using combination chakra acupuncture, the Key points need to be stimulated first, followed by the needling and sedation of the chakra and meridian source points. Many of the points are bilateral, so a fair number of needles need to be inserted at the same time. If, however, you do not wish to needle every peripheral point bilaterally, it does not lessen the treatment's affect. Also, using this method, there is never an instant or miraculous improvement in the symptoms. Because it is the chakra energies that are being addressed, it takes time for healing (by the patient) to take place. Please be aware of and make your patient aware of the need for healing time. There is no doubt, in my opinion, that this way of treating chronic conditions with acupuncture produces a quicker and more long-lasting alternative to traditional Chinese acupuncture.

In the following, the needling for each combination is shown with an example of a condition within the scope of that particular combination. Each shows one formula of treatment with acupuncture. When using combination chakra acupuncture, the time required is slightly longer than when using the major or minor chakras individually—allow approximately half an hour for each formula (Figures 4.1 to 4.6).

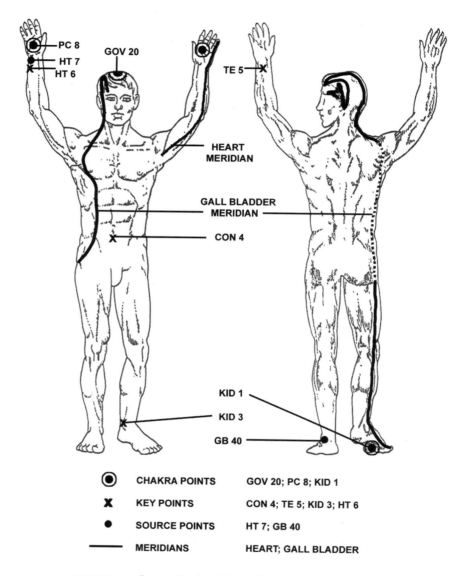

PC 8
GOV 20
HT 7
HT 6
TE 5

HEART
MERIDIAN

GALL BLADDER
MERIDIAN

CON 4

KID 1
KID 3
GB 40

⊙	CHAKRA POINTS	GOV 20; PC 8; KID 1
X	KEY POINTS	CON 4; TE 5; KID 3; HT 6
●	SOURCE POINTS	HT 7; GB 40
—	MERIDIANS	HEART; GALL BLADDER

FIGURE 4.1. *Crown, Hand, and Foot Chakra Combination Points*

CROWN, HAND, AND FOOT CONDITIONS

For example: Vertigo

1. Stimulate the Key points—Con 4, TE 5, HT 6, and KID 3.
2. Sedate the chakra points—Gov 20, PC 8, and KID 1.

3. Sedate the meridian Source points—HT 7 and GB 40.

4. Stimulate the Key points for a few seconds every five minutes and leave all needles in situ for approximately thirty minutes.

BROW, GROIN, AND CLAVICULAR CONDITIONS

For example: Migraine

1. Stimulate the Key points—Gov 4, SP 6, PC 7, and LR 8.

2. Sedate the chakra points—Extra 1 *(Yintang)*, ST 30, and KID 27.

3. Sedate the meridian Source points—PC 7 and ST 42.

4. Stimulate the Key points for a few seconds every five minutes and leave all needles *in situ* for approximately thirty minutes.

Please remember that PC 7 is a Key point *and* a Source point, and therefore does not need to be needled twice!

THROAT, SHOULDER, AND NAVEL CONDITIONS

For example: Chronic Bronchitis

1. Stimulate the Key points—Con 6, LR 5, ST 40, and LI 11.

2. Sedate the chakra points—Con 22, LI 15, and KID 16.

3. Sedate the meridian Source points—LU 9 and LI 4.

4. Stimulate the Key points for a few seconds every five minutes and leave all needles *in situ* for approximately thirty minutes.

HEART, EAR, AND INTERCOSTAL CONDITIONS

For example: Thoracic Shingles

1. Stimulate the Key points—Gov 7, HT 1, TE 4, and GB 37.

2. Sedate the chakra points—Con 17, TE 17, and SP 21.

3. Sedate the meridian Source points—SP 3 and TE 4.

4. Stimulate the Key points for a few seconds every five minutes and leave all needles *in situ* for approximately thirty minutes.

Please note that acupoint TE 4 is a Key point *and* Source point so need not be treated twice.

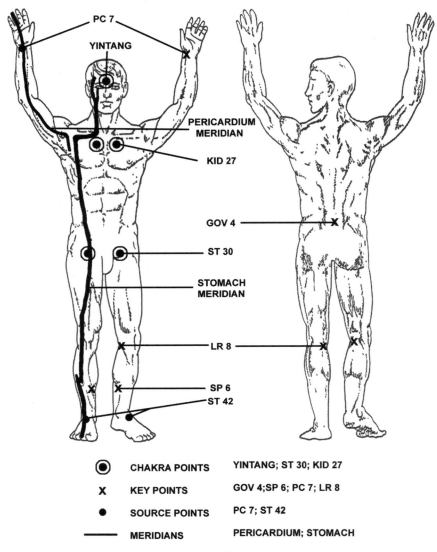

FIGURE 4.2. *Brow, Clavicular, and Groin Chakra Combination Points*

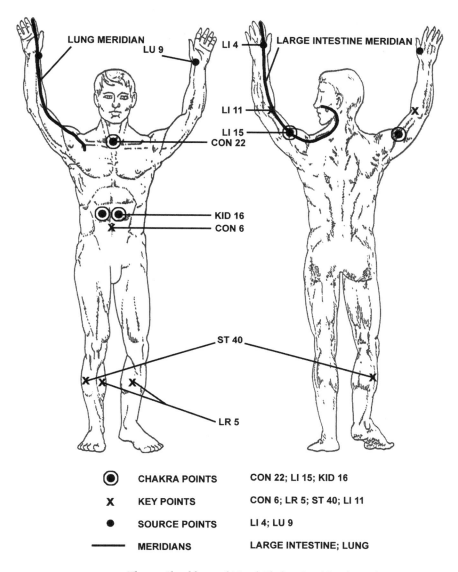

FIGURE 4.3. *Throat, Shoulder, and Navel Chakra Combination Points*

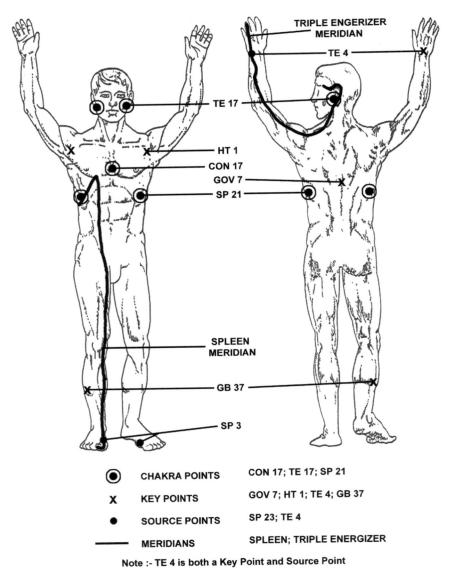

◉ CHAKRA POINTS	CON 17; TE 17; SP 21	
X KEY POINTS	GOV 7; HT 1; TE 4; GB 37	
● SOURCE POINTS	SP 23; TE 4	
—— MERIDIANS	SPLEEN; TRIPLE ENERGIZER	

Note :- TE 4 is both a Key Point and Source Point

FIGURE 4.4. *Heart, Ear, and Intercostal Chakra Combination Points*

SOLAR PLEXUS, SACRAL, AND SPLEEN CONDITIONS

For example: Chronic Fatigue Syndrome

1. Stimulate the Key points—Con 17, TE 4, Gov 12, PC 3, and Gov 8.

2. Sedate the chakra points—Con 14, Con 6, and SP 16 (L).

3. Sedate the meridian Source points—LR 3 and SI 4.

4. Stimulate the Key points for a few seconds every five minutes and leave all needles *in situ* for approximately thirty minutes.

BASE, ELBOW, AND KNEE CONDITIONS

For example: Spinal Arthritis

1. Stimulate the Key points—Con 22, LR 8, BL 59, and SI 7.

2. Sedate the chakra points—Con 2, PC 3, and BL 40.

3. Sedate the meridian Source points—KID 3 and BL 64.

4. Stimulate the Key points for a few seconds every five minutes and leave all needles *in situ* for approximately thirty minutes.

The above treatments represent a breakthrough in the treatment of chronic disease. My own experience of using these methods has shown that the number of treatment sessions required to substantially improve the health of these patients has dramatically reduced when compared to traditional acupuncture. Even though this type of acupuncture is new to the vast majority of readers and would seem a rather strange paradigm, all that is asked of you is to try it! Use *Acupuncture and the Chakra Energy System* as a practical workbook, and you will be amazed. Feedback through my website—www.johncrossclinics.com—is always welcome.

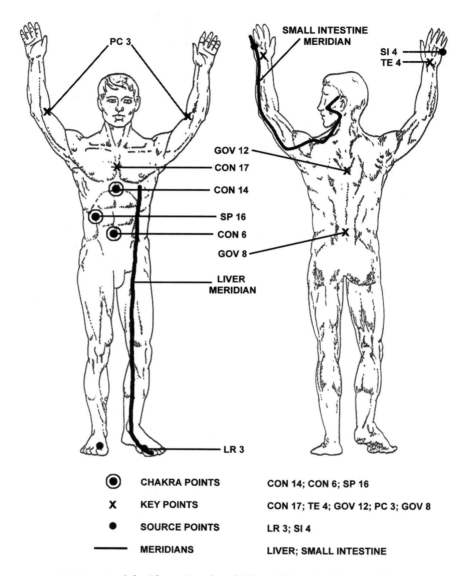

⊙	CHAKRA POINTS	CON 14; CON 6; SP 16
X	KEY POINTS	CON 17; TE 4; GOV 12; PC 3; GOV 8
●	SOURCE POINTS	LR 3; SI 4
——	MERIDIANS	LIVER; SMALL INTESTINE

FIGURE 4.5. *Solar Plexus, Sacral, and Spleen Chakra Combination Points*

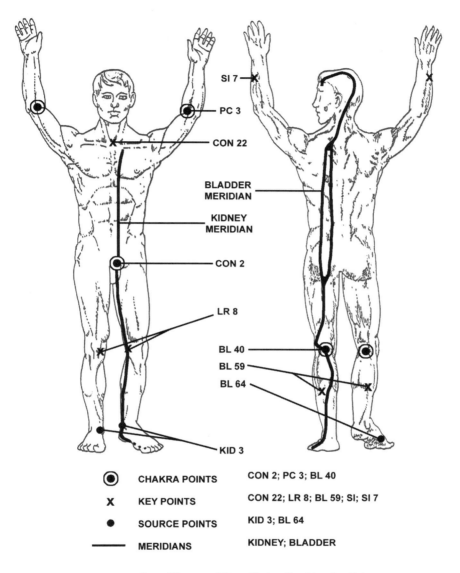

FIGURE 4.6. *Base, Elbow, and Knee Chakra Combination Points*

HORMONAL PRODUCTION USING THE MAJOR CHAKRAS, THE EIGHT EXTRAORDINARY MERIDIANS, AND BLADDER 1

The use of the key points of the eight extra (extraordinary) meridians together with a few other acupoints in the production of hormonal secretions has been known for a number of years. My research has found that hormonal production may be enhanced in a remarkable way by using the major chakras, the key points of the eight extraordinary meridians, and acupoint Bladder 1. Bladder 1 (BL 1) is one of those points with which acupuncturists seem to have a love-hate relationship. The point is situated one-tenth of a cun lateral and superior to the inner canthus of the eye near the medial orbital border. Many acupuncturists hate to use this influential point because it is so close to the eye, and even if used correctly it can cause internal bruising which may give the appearance of a black eye. Although the traditional texts state that the point is used for dispelling internal wind and eliminating heat, it is generally agreed that stimulation of the point affects the anterior pituitary gland, hence its association with hormonal production. If you can use this point with ease, you should carry on using it. To the majority of you who do not wish to use it, there is an alternative. BL 1 is very close to the anterior aspect of the Brow chakra and produces a similar influence. Therefore, to produce the same affect as using BL 1, the Key points of the Brow chakra should be stimulated, followed by needling *Yintang* (Extra 1), which is the acupoint of the anterior Brow chakra. The points used are therefore Gov 4, SP 6, and *Yintang*. In this section of the chapter whenever BL 1 is mentioned, the three substitute points may be used with equal effect. The hormonal productions discussed are adrenaline, cortisone, thyroxine, and sex hormones (Figures 4.7 relates).

ADRENALINE

Adrenaline is produced by the adrenal (suprarenal) medulla. Under quiet resting conditions the blood contains very little adrenaline. During excitement or circumstances that demand special effort, adrenaline is released into the blood stream. Adrenaline constricts the smooth muscle of the

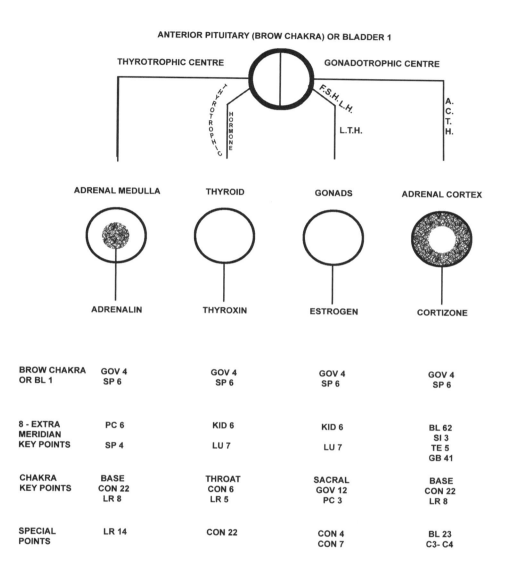

FIGURE 4.7. *Hormonal Production using the Chakras, Key Points, and Bladder 1*

skin which makes the hairs stand on end and produce "goose flesh." Adrenaline dilates the pupils of the eye to admit more light, dilates the blood vessels of the heart and skeletal muscles to give a rich supply of oxygenated blood in case of emergencies, raises the blood pressure, dilates the bronchus and bronchioles, stimulates metabolism, and increases blood coagulation properties. The common denominator in all these functions is that it directly stimulates the sympathetic nervous system.

The adrenal medulla may be controlled by the Base chakra—a combination of *Chong Mai, Yin Wei Mai,* and Bladder 1. Special point LR 14 is also used. The conditions where natural adrenaline would be required would be those with a weakened sympathetic nerve outflow. Examples of these are:

- Congestive heart conditions
- Intermittent claudication
- Chronic asthma
- Cramps
- Pre performance treatment for premier athletes

ORDER OF TREATMENT (see Figures 4.8 and 4.7 for pictorial form)

1. Stimulate Bladder 1 *or* Extra 1, Gov 4, and SP 6 (Brow chakra).
2. Stimulate PC 6 and SP 4 (Key points of *Chong Mai* and *Yin Wei Mai*).
3. Stimulate Con 22 and LR 8 (Key points of Base chakra).
4. Needle Con 2 (Base chakra point).
5. The special point of LR 14 is sometimes used.

I have used the adrenaline technique many times when treating chronic asthma, obtaining excellent results each time. Do not be afraid of overstimulation. The human body balances naturally—you will not make your patient high. Please remember it is the patient's natural adrenaline that is being produced, not the synthetic chemical sometimes injected into patients to treat asthma. Your patients should be warned that they will be quite tired for the remainder of the day. The fatigue is a natural reaction to treatment, so your patient should rest afterward—discourage fighting this fatigue in any way.

Hormones

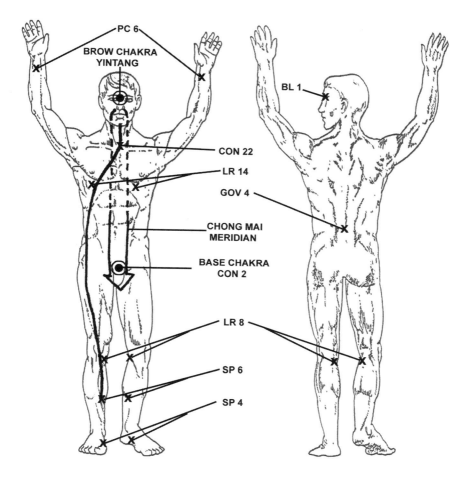

FIGURE 4.8. *Acupoints in Adrenaline Production*

THYROXINE

Thyroxine is produced by the thyroid gland. It is a combination hormone comprising of triiodothyronine hormone and tetraiodothyronine hormone. These active hormones are released by the thyroid gland into general circulation for distribution by the blood stream to all body tissues where they act as catalysts hastening the oxidation processes in tissue cells. Thyroxine also regulates the various enzymes which control energy metabolism and thus influences metabolic processes.

The thyroid is controlled by the Throat chakra, a combination of *Ren Mai* (Conception), *Yinchiao Mai,* and Bladder 1. Conditions where the patient would require the natural production of thyroxine would include:

- Extreme physical fatigue
- Growth retardation
- Feeling cold all the time
- Reduced appetite coupled with weight gain
- Mental fatigue or inability to think clearly

ORDER OF TREATMENT (see Figures 4.9 and Figure 4.7)
1. Stimulate Bladder 1 (or the Brow chakra points).
2. Stimulate KID 6 and LU 7 (Key points of *Yinchiao Mai* and *Ren Mai*).
3. Stimulate Con 6 and LR 5 (Key points of the Throat chakra).
4. Needle Con 22 (Throat chakra point).

The thyroid treatment will require several sessions but is well worth pursuing. Patients often report the immediate health improvements, such as having energy (weight loss takes longer to achieve and must be executed with a sensible, calorie-controlled eating plan).

FEMALE SEX HORMONES
(PROGESTERONE AND ESTROGEN)

Estrogen and progesterone are produced by the uterus and put into the circulation to maintain a normal menstrual cycle. Estrogen is produced during the first half of the cycle and both are produced during the second half. They are also produced during puberty to ensure that the primary and secondary sexual characteristics form. The sex hormones are controlled by the Sacral chakra, a combination of *Yinchiao Mai, Ren Mai,* and Bladder 1. Special points Con 4 and Con 7 may also be used. A breakdown in the production of these two hormones may lead to the following conditions:

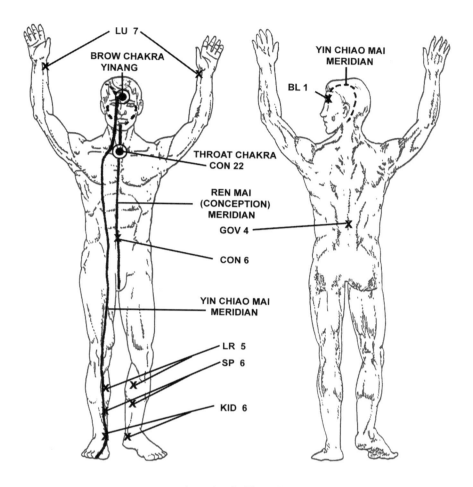

FIGURE 4.9. *Acupoints in Thyroxine Production*

• Dysmenorrhea
• Amenorrhea
• Menopausal symptoms
• Pre-menstrual symptoms (physical and emotional)
• Painful breasts

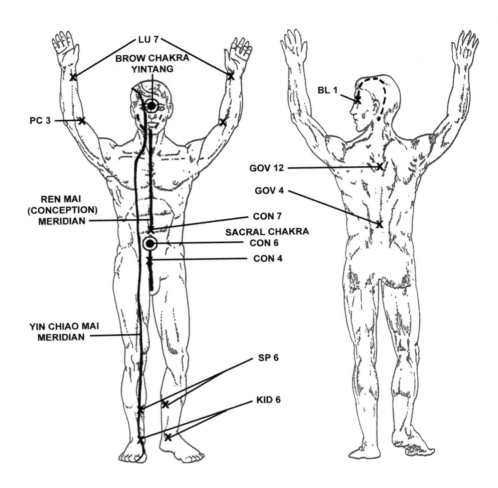

FIGURE 4.10. *Acupoints in Female Sex Hormones Production*

ORDER OF TREATMENT (see Figures 4.10 and 4.7 for pictorial form)

1. Stimulate Bladder 1 (or the Brow chakra).

2. Stimulate KID 6 and LU 7 (Key points *Yinchiao Mai* and *Ren Mai*)

3. Stimulate Con 4 and Con 7 (special points)

4. Stimulate PC 3 and Gov 12 (Key points of Sacral chakra)

5. Needle Con 6 (Sacral chakra point)

I cannot recall the number of times I have used this formula for treating the most intransigent of menstrual imbalances, but it must be over two hundred. An example will be presented in the Case Histories section later in this chapter.

CORTISONE

Cortisone is produced by the adrenal cortex. Under-activity of cortisone produces a fall in blood sodium level and a rise in blood potassium level, giving rise to the following:

- Muscular wasting and weakness
- Gastrointestinal upsets
- Anemia
- Pigmentation
- Low blood sugar
- Rheumatoid conditions
- Tightness of the chest wall and breathing difficulties

Over-activity of cortisone produces the opposite cellular activity and can give rise to:

- Edema (excess fluid in the tissues)
- Cushing's disease
- Secondary sex characteristics, such as female facial hair, etc.

The adrenal cortex (and subsequently the natural production of cortisone) is controlled by the Base chakra, *Du Mai* (Governor channel), *Yangchiao Mai, Yangwei Mai, Dai mai,* Bladder 1, the special point BL 23, and the non-meridian acupoint between C3 and C4.

ORDER OF TREATMENT (see Figures 4.11 and 4.7 for pictorial form)

1. Stimulate Bladder 1 (or the Brow chakra points).
2. Stimulate BL 62 and SI 3 (Key points of the *Du Mai* and *Yangchiao Mai*).

3. Stimulate TE 5 and GB 41 (Key points of *Yangwei Mai* and *Dai Mai*).

4. Stimulate the special points of BL 23 and the acupoint between C3-4.

5. Stimulate Con 22 and LR 8 (Key points of the Base chakra).

6. Needle Con 2 (Base chakra point).

The cortisone order of treatment may seem, at the outset, to use an awful lot of needles. In fact, no more needles are used than in a traditional approach to such difficult and chronic conditions. To be able to help a patient produce his or her own cortisone is a prize that is worth more than gold. This treatment does *not* represent a one needle and one treatment wonder. It requires significant work on the part of the practitioner. The reward for the accomplishment of cortisone acupuncture treatment for both patient and practitioner is significant.

During this chapter, concentration has been on the treatment of chronic conditions. Acute conditions can usually be addressed by other acupuncture modalities. You, the acupuncturist, may make a couple of observations when reading this chapter. First you may observe that more acupoints are needled as part of a more complicated procedure than with the tried and tested methods that you have used in the past: this is sometimes, but not always true. Secondly, you may observe that TCM has a treatment for every ailment, and therefore may conclude that learning a different acupuncture modality may prove unnecessary. These two and several similar thought processes have been presented to me over the years. The importance of learning my new method of treatment can be understood through the lens of the underlying philosophy of that work. Chakra acupuncture is *not* a branch of TCM: the philosophy is different, although many Chakra acupuncture ideas are associated with TCM. Chakra acupuncture represents the energy balance and treatment of the real *cause* of a condition by affecting the Physical, Etheric, Emotional, and Mental pathways of pure vital force. The cause of the condition is being addressed, not just the ensuing symptoms. Further, you will find that your patient will require fewer visits in order to achieve the desired results. If you are

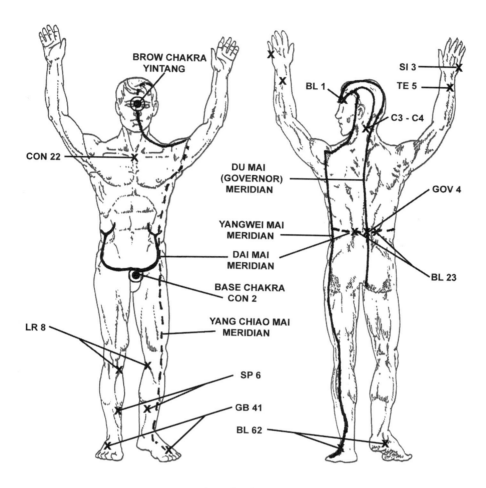

FIGURE 4.11. *Acupoints in Cortisone Production*

in private practice you may need to adjust compensation accordingly, but otherwise may find yourself content to be compensated with the joy you will bring to your patient. However, do not get carried away with the idea that these chakra acupuncture techniques are miraculous or instant. Remember that *no* medicine, save perhaps divine healing, can reverse that which is physiologically irreversible, so please do not think that you can cure the incurable.

TREATMENT OF TEN NAMED CONDITIONS USING CHAKRA ACUPUNCTURE

The following ten conditions represent a cross section of the conditions that you are likely to encounter. The word "named" is purposely used because if you were treating conditions using traditional philosophy, they would not have a Western name that we as practitioners understand. Each condition (or polyglot of symptoms) would be given a traditional translation that would best describe what is occurring within the emotions and body (psycho and soma). Examples of these would be "Liver damp rising," "Sacral chakra congestion," "Shen energy imbalance," and so on. By using Western terminology, we are all "singing from the same hymn sheet." Having said that, it is important that you as the practitioner understand that it is the *person* who happens to have certain energy imbalances who is treated, *not* the condition itself. Named conditions may have several different causes, and it is always the individual etiology that must be addressed—hence the beauty and efficacy of the chakra energy system in treating causes.

The ten named conditions are as follows:

- Chronic sore throats and colds
- Asthma
- Insomnia
- Chronic lower back pain
- Dysmenorrhea
- Rheumatoid arthritis
- Psoriasis
- Depression and Anxiety
- Frozen shoulder
- Hypertension

CHRONIC SORE THROATS AND COLDS

These can be a disabling conditions that affect people of all ages and not just children. There is no one simple cause. Possible causes are:

1. In children and adolescents, the Throat chakra becomes congested by the attempt to purge accumulated toxins. Constipation often accompanies this affliction.

2. In adults, the Throat chakra becomes over-active in people unable to express themselves in thought, will, or deed. This chakra is also affected by sudden emotional shock.

3. When the tonsils have been removed in children and adults (and the first line of defense in bacterial invasion has disappeared), a congestion of the Throat chakra will result with the sacral chakra possibly involved.

4. As a possible secondary affect of sexual imbalances that affect the sacral chakra and causes the Throat chakra to become under-stimulated or over-stimulated.

AIMS OF TREATMENT

The aim of treatment is to obtain an energy balance at the Throat chakra and, where applicable, the Sacral chakra.

METHOD OF TREATMENT

The easiest method of treatment is to use the combination of major and minor chakras that are associated with the throat region, i.e., Throat, Shoulder, and Navel combination. The associated meridians with this combination are the Lung and Large Intestine, both linked to organs of excretion which provide the perfect way to purge toxins as the patient begins to detoxify. The patient must be warned that even after the first session they may experience a worse sore throat, diarrhea, or a mild rash. They should be instructed not to take any suppressive medication. The acupoints Con 6, LR 5, ST 40, and LI 11 (Key points) are stimulated for a few seconds every five minutes. In addition, Con 22, Gov 14. LI 15, and KID 16 (major and minor chakra points) are needled and left *in situ* for approximately twenty to thirty minutes (sedated). Points need not be used bilaterally. The patient must be kept warm but ventilated during treatment. Subsequent treatments will probably follow the same procedure but in my experience this condition rarely requires more than three sessions.

Asthma

Asthma is a complicated condition. Orthodox medicine gives many causes of asthma ranging from bacteria to stress. When doing chakra acupuncture, the actual cause of the imbalance means very little, because the imbalance or weakness that is causing the disease *(dis-ease)* will be put right at source of the problem, which is almost always emotional. People with asthma and many other conditions with emotional etiology respond very well to chakra acupuncture treatments.

AIMS OF TREATMENT

The aim of treatment is to balance the most affected chakras, which are the Throat and Heart. Sometimes with asthma that is impure, the patient exhibits some allergic and eczema tendencies, creating a need to balance the Solar Plexus chakra.

METHOD OF TREATMENT

The treatment of choice is to balance and treat the Throat and Heart chakras, then utilize other modalities such as reflexology and Bach (homeopathic) remedies as on-going medication. Acupoints used in order are:

1. To balance and treat the Throat chakra, stimulate the Key points of Con 6 and LR 5, followed by sedation of the Throat and Sacral chakra (coupled chakra) points—Con 22, Gov 14, and Con 6. Please note that Con 6 is both the Key point of the Throat chakra and the Sacral chakra acupoint—therefore it needs to be stimulated initially and then left *in situ.*

2. To balance and treat the Heart chakra, stimulate the Key points of HT 1 and Gov 7, followed by sedation of the Heart chakra and Solar plexus chakra (couple)—Con 17, Gov 10 and Con 14. Needles are placed *in situ* as before. A soothing pattern of reflexology is helpful following the acupuncture. There is no need for the usual points LI 4 and LU 7. The minor chakras are not required either. Please note that some authorities consider acupoint HT 1

to be forbidden—use it with care and only if experienced and trained in the procedure.

INSOMNIA

Insomnia has many causes. The ideal approach to insomnia is to treat the known cause, but this is often difficult to ascertain if there is an ongoing stressful situation in the patient's home or work environment. However, by using this powerful form of acupuncture, the astral (emotional) level of the patient can be addressed. Often, but not always, the Brow and Heart chakras are the ones that require energy balancing.

AIMS OF TREATMENT

The aim of treatment is to balance the Brow and Heart chakras and their associated meridians of Gall Bladder, Heart, and Small Intestine.

METHOD OF TREATMENT

1. To balance and treat the Brow chakra, stimulate the Key points—Gov 4 and SP 6, followed by sedation of the Brow chakra and Base chakra (couple) points—Extra 1 *(Yintang)*, Gov 16, and Con 2.

2. To balance and treat the Heart chakra, stimulate the Key points of HT 1 and GOV 7, followed by sedation of the Heart chakra and Solar Plexus chakra (couple) points—Con 17, Gov 10, and Con 14.

3. To stimulate the associated meridians, stimulate the Source points of the Gall Bladder, Heart, and Small Intestine meridians—GB 40, HT 7, and SI 4.

4. Teach the patient the best trick of getting off to sleep when the mind is racing: hold the anterior Brow chakra point at Extra 1 *(Yintang)* with the middle finger pad of one hand and HT 7 with the other middle finger while lying on one's side. I have made many life-long friends by teaching this simple self-help method to people who are desperate for a good night of sleep.

Chronic Lower Back Pain

More research has been carried out and more money spent on the causes and treatment of lower back pain than any other musculo-skeletal condition. More sick days are due to lower back pain than the common cold. There are as many types of bad backs as there are people who are suffering from it. In other words, each person should be treated as an individual. The pain part of the condition may be treated very effectively with traditional, Western, or minor chakra acupuncture. The real cause of the pain could be as diverse as poor diet, poor posture, a previous injury (such as a fall on to the coccyx), or a kidney condition. Why, I hear you ask, would a poor diet be a contributing factor to a chronic lumbar condition? Chinese medicine states that the ligaments and soft tissue are ruled by the Spleen and the Stomach. Thus, the supporting ligaments can become congested and weak due to many years of eating denatured foods. In addition, the most common level to be affected is the Lumbar 4-5 junction. The Lumbar 4-5 area is related to the large intestine (sympathetic nerve supply and lymphatic drainage region according to Applied Kinesiology). My first book *Acupressure—Clinical Applications in Musculo-Skeletal Conditions* taught the use of acupressure in musculo-skeletal conditions, and a whole section dealt with the influence of chemical and emotional etiology that cause seemingly mechanical conditions.

AIMS OF TREATMENT

Treatment aims to energy balance and treat the Base chakra together with its minor chakra counterparts (Knee and Elbow) in pain relief. The stomach, spleen, and liver meridians are also involved (ligaments and soft tissue).

METHOD OF TREATMENT

1. To balance and treat the Base chakra, stimulate the Key points— LR 8 and Con 22, followed by sedation of the Base and Crown (couple) chakra points—Con 2, Gov 2, and Gov 20.

2. To use Schedule Two minor chakra pain relief points (see Chapter Three), stimulate Key points of the Knee and Elbow chakras—

BL 59 and SI 7, followed by sedation of the Elbow and Knee chakra points—PC3 and BL 40.

3. The Stomach, Spleen, and Liver meridian Source points should now be stimulated—ST 42, SP 3, and LR 3.

The Base chakra treatment I have presented here is radically different from the usual acupuncture treatment for this condition. Even though I have used these methods for over thirty years without additional acupoints, it may help psychologically if your patient experiences you performing some localized acupuncture to the lumbar spine at the same time. Lying on the side may be the position of choice in order to entertain both Conception and Governor acupoints at the same time.

DYSMENORRHEA

The gynecological condition of dysmenorrhea may be greatly helped with chakra acupuncture. Pre-menstrual girls and older women are sometimes afflicted with this condition. The causes are complex and may include hormonal imbalance and a lumbo-sacral condition with referral of imbalance from the spine to the uterus. The majority of cases will respond to the balancing and treatment of the Sacral chakra.

AIMS OF TREATMENT

The aim of dysmenorrhea treatment is to energy balance and treat the Sacral chakra. In patients who exhibit a great deal of pain, using Schedule Three for minor chakra pain relief formula is required (see Chapter Three for details).

METHOD OF TREATMENT

1. To energy balance and treat the Sacral chakra, stimulate the Key points of Gov 12 and PC 3, followed by the sedation of the Sacral and Throat (couple) chakra points—Con 6 and Con 22 (add the posterior aspect of the Sacral chakra—Gov 3 between L4-5 if a spinal nerve root referral is thought to be the cause).

2. To use Schedule Three minor chakra pain relief points, stimulate the Key points of the Groin and Clavicular chakras—PC 7 and LR 8, followed by sedation of the Groin and Clavicular chakra points—ST 30 and KID 27.

RHEUMATOID ARTHRITIS

The disabling condition rheumatoid arthritis may be seen in the acute, sub-acute, and chronic stages. Chronic rheumatoid arthritis (RA) answers best to chakra acupuncture. The etiology is often complicated, but the latest research indicates bacteriological involvement. Typically, a strong genetic predisposition for full-blown RA exists in a patient for RA to develop, even though millions of people possess the rheumatoid "factor" in their genetic coding. The trigger causing a person to go from simply having the rheumatoid factor to having RA is often a shock to the system such as a physical accident or a sudden grief.

AIMS OF TREATMENT

Rheumatoid arthritis treatment aims to energy balance the Base and Sacral chakras and liberates cortisone in chronic cases (see earlier in this chapter for details).

METHOD OF TREATMENT

1. To balance and treat the Base chakra, stimulate the Key points—Con 22 and LR 8, followed by sedation of the Base and Crown (couple) chakra points—Con 2, Gov 2, and Gov 20.

2. To balance and treat the Sacral chakra, stimulate the Key points—Gov 12 and PC 3, followed by sedation of the Sacral and Throat (couple) chakra points—Con 6 and Con 22 (please note that Con 22 is the anterior Throat chakra acupoint as well as being one of the two Key points of the Base chakra).

3. Using the cortisone-liberating formula—Stimulate BL 1 (or the Brow chakra), BL 62, SI 3, TE 5, and GB 41. Followed by the

stimulation of special points BL 23 and the acupoint between C3 and C4. The final points in this part of the treatment—Con 22, LR 8, and Con 2 have already been treated as the needles will still be *in situ*.

It may be difficult for your rheumatoid patient to lie prone, so any point on the back such as Gov 2, Gov 12, and BL 23 should be carried out with the patient either lying on his or her side or sitting at the end of the session. With any condition where lying down is difficult, sitting may be used as an alternate position. Subsequent sessions may not require the cortisone-liberating part of the treatment.

PSORIASIS

Psoriasis is a very disturbing skin condition and is one of the most difficult conditions to treat successfully. Psoriasis is a highly complex condition of the rheumatoid taint, but is primarily the result of a Solar Plexus chakra imbalance. Because of its chronicity, the Base chakra has to be addressed as well. The treatment outlined below indicates the best solution that I have discovered. I have used this treatment for years on scores of patients with this condition with success.

AIMS OF TREATMENT

The aim of Psoriasis treatment is to energy balance and treat the Base chakra and the Solar Plexus, Sacral, and Spleen combination.

METHOD OF TREATMENT

1. To energy balance and treat the Base chakra—stimulate the Key points—Con 22 and LR 8, followed by sedating the Base and Crown (couple) chakra points—Con 2, Gov 2, and Gov 20

2. To use the combination approach of Solar Plexus/Sacral/Spleen— stimulate the Key points—Con 17, TE 4, Gov 12, PC 3, and Gov 8, followed by sedation of the chakra acupoints—Con 14, Con 6, and SP 16.

The method outlined may seem to be a complicated way of treating this condition, but experience has shown that psoriasis shows remarkable intransigent qualities and requires a heavy treatment to attempt to cure it. As with every skin condition, remind the patient that, even after the first session, there could be a time after treatment when the skin appears to be worse. The patient will be very tempted to use more suppressive medications in the form of cortisone-based ointments, but this should be dissuaded at all costs. Simple emulsifying ointments such as aqueous cream should be used to soothe the skin as the treatment attempts to get the patient to heal themselves from the inside out.

DEPRESSION AND ANXIETY

Acupuncture has been used more frequently in recent years for the symptoms of depression and anxiety. Even though traditional Chinese acupuncture has a good track record of easing symptoms in emotional conditions, it does not address the causes. By using chakra acupuncture, the etiology of the emotional imbalance will be addressed. If the Heart and Solar Plexus chakras are balanced and treated, this will satisfy many types of both anxiety and depression. These two conditions often arise because of worry about another disease. It is said that, "It is not so much disease itself that destroys, but the *thought* of the disease that produces havoc within the economy." This gnomic statement is particularly true for a serious illness such as cancer. The Heart chakra is used as it deals with any condition that affects the emotions and psyche. The Solar Plexus chakra is used because of its role in the dissemination of waste (thoughts included). These two major chakras happen to be coupled chakras, so the two are often treated together.

AIMS OF TREATMENT

Depression and anxiety treatment aims to energy balance and treat the Heart and Solar Plexus chakras.

METHODS OF TREATMENT

The Heart and Solar Plexus chakras may be treated at the same time. This is done by stimulating the Key points of Gov 7, HT 1, and TE 4. The other Solar Plexus chakra Key point—Con 17 is also the acupoint of the Heart chakra, so this needs to be sedated in this instance following the initial stimulation. These four points are immediately followed by sedating the Heart and Solar Plexus chakra points of Con 14 (and Con 17). An adjunct point that may be used is the ear point *Shenmen.* While the needles are *in situ,* it is excellent to carry out some light touch reflexology where the same reflected chakras would be targeted.

FROZEN SHOULDER

The disabling condition Frozen Shoulder may have several causes. The obvious cause is mechanical, the result of a direct blow to the shoulder girdle area or lower cervical region. The most common cause of Frozen Shoulder, however, is a combination of faulty eating and other toxic build-up around the tissues of the shoulder girdle. The condition may be the result of the body's attempt to rid itself of toxins on a physical and emotional level. If this is the case, it is often accompanied with constipation, catarrh, and mild depression. Experience has told me that the best way to treat Frozen Shoulder is by balancing the Heart chakra (only if it is *not* a mechanical cause) and by using the combination chakras of Throat, Shoulder, and Navel (for mechanical, emotional, or toxic etiology). The Heart chakra regime I am describing will treat the emotional and physical pain of this condition.

AIMS OF TREATMENT

The aim of Frozen Shoulder treatment is to energy balance and treat the Heart chakra and the combination of Throat, Shoulder, and Navel.

METHOD OF TREATMENT

1. To energy balance and treat the Heart chakra, stimulate the Key points Gov 7 and HT 1, followed by sedation of the Heart and Solar Plexus (couple) chakra points—Con 17 and Con 14.

2. To use the combination of Throat, Shoulder, and Navel chakras, stimulate the Key points—Con 6, LR 5, ST 40, and LI 11. This is followed by sedation of the chakra points—Con 22, Gov 14, LI 15, and KID 16.

Coupling acupuncture treatment with a gentle exercise regime and passive movement (never forced) will help considerably. The patient should be encouraged to do some gentle "pendulum" home exercises and to swim regularly. Pendulum exercises consist of leaning forward with the arm swinging freely, taking it through flexion, extension, abduction, and circular movement. These exercises are most effective when executed with a small counter weight in the hand. Frozen shoulder is a condition that may have a strong emotional etiology and often resolves while the patient cries on the couch. Once emotional release has occurred, it is amazing how quickly the shoulder resolves itself. Keep a box of tissues handy!

HYPERTENSION

Regardless of the cause of hypertension (which is merely a symptom of other imbalances in the body) the classical chakra acupuncture treatment I have used successfully for several years of using the Crown, Hand, and Foot combination works effectively.

AIMS OF TREATMENT

The aim of hypertension treatment is to energy balance and treat the system using the Crown, Hand, and Foot combination.

METHOD OF TREATMENT

To use the Crown, Hand, and Foot combination, stimulate the Key points—Con 4, TE 5, HT 6, and KID 3. This is followed by sedation of the chakra points—Gov 20, PC 8, and KID 1. Be careful to monitor the blood pressure prior to and after treatment and do not sit the patient up too quickly following treatment. The patient should be ordered to rest as much as possible following the session. This treatment regimen should be repeated on a weekly basis until the blood pressure has stabilized over a period of time.

CASE HISTORIES

The following Case Histories have been added to give the reader a more personal and in-depth practical understanding of this type of acupuncture therapy. Each one is genuine (with the names changed) and represents a cross-section of conditions that I have treated over the past twenty-five years.

Lower Back Pain with Sciatica

HISTORY

Geoffrey was a forty-five-year-old car mechanic who had been troubled with lower back pain for the previous ten years. The most problematic action he could do was to constantly bend over the hood of a car. He found that it was difficult to straighten up after about ten minutes of bending over the hood. The only time he could recall hurting his back was when he had fallen heavily on his coccyx as a child. He had tried physical therapy, chiropractic alignment, and massage in the previous five years. Each therapy had helped slightly but the sciatica had always returned. He also told me that he suffered from irritable bowel syndrome (IBS) which affected him at work.

EXAMINATION

An examination revealed that Geoffrey had lumbo-sacral spasm and pain with sciatic referral of the right leg down to the lateral aspect of the ankle. The pain was constant and made worse for movement and better for rest. Some analgesics helped, but only for a short period.

FIRST TREATMENT SESSION

Even though Geoffrey had suffered for ten years, I decided to treat the condition as an acute one and used the minor chakra pain relief points.

He was quite happy to receive acupuncture as he had not experienced it before and had tried "everything else." The main area of pain was situated in the lower lumbar spine which corresponded to Schedule Two of the Pain Relief Areas. The Key points of BL 59 and SI 7 were inserted bilaterally and stimulated every five minutes for approximately half and hour. The minor chakra points of BL 40 and PC 3 were inserted shortly after the Key points and were left *in situ* without any stimulation (save that of achieving *de qui*). In such cases, you may be tempted to insert needles locally in the lumbar spine and BL 62 under the lateral malleolus as you would probably do with TCM—please do not do this as it will defeat the object of using this new technique. After half an hour of comfortable lying prone the needles were removed and after about five minutes he dressed and left the surgery. There was an obvious look of disappointment on his face. I asked to see him a week later and advised him to keep the spine warm and as flexible as discomfort allowed (he was on vacation for a week so he was not working).

SECOND TREATMENT SESSION

Geoffrey arrived for his second session with a huge grin on his face. The evening of the treatment had been very painful, and he had been forced to take more pain killers. He had woken up the next morning feeling much better, and the improvement in his condition continued throughout the week. He had not tested his spine by doing any exercises or hard labor. His sciatica was still there, but it was of lesser intensity and was now only down to the back of the thigh. Geoffrey had noticed that he had slight discomfort around the lower sacral and coccyx region (As a basic naturopathic response, a lesion often creates deep bruising at the site of the original trauma). Because his body responded so well to the first treatment of the minor chakras, I decided to do the same treatment again. Since the discomfort had shifted lower down the spine into the Schedule Three area, it is this Schedule that was treated. The Key points of PC 7 and LR 8 were inserted and stimulated like the last time. The minor chakra points of ST 30 and KID 27 were also needled. He was in supine lying down for the session and this time was not at all puzzled as to why the lower spine had not been needled—he just accepted it. I taught him inner-range spinal strengthening exercises—consisting of him prone lying and gently raising the shoulders and feet off the ground to a count of five. I asked him to telephone after a further week. He reported the next week in fine health with no re-occurrence of back pain or sciatica in the following week when he had been working. I saw him once more three months later for a check-up. He was delighted that his irritable bowel syndrome (IBS) had "miraculously" eased.

MENOPAUSAL HOT FLASHES

Debbie was a fifty-four-year-old single woman who had had severe hot flashes since her menopause that had started seven years previously. She had been on hormonal replacement therapy without success. Debbie had tried many different herbal and homeopathic remedies to ease the symptoms, but she could not cure herself this way. She was a secretary by profession and was finding life increasingly embarrassing in that she always needed to cool down and take breaks away from the office. Her night sweats had become extreme. Apart from herbal treatments she had tried reflexology, which, although it made the symptoms less severe, by making her less anxious—she still suffered immensely. She telephoned me following a conversation with her neighbor who had consulted me with a similar problem.

HISTORY

Debbie had been relatively free from illness for most of her life, having few or no menstrual symptoms. However, she had suffered from the occasional debilitating migraine. Her digestion was also suspect since she could not ingest pastries or other sugar-laden substances without having indigestion. The hot flashes affected her whole body and were worse at night when she was often forced to change the sweat-soaked sheets.

FIRST TREATMENT SESSION

From the history, abdominal analysis, tongue analysis, and pulse, I decided to energy balance and treat the Sacral chakra—the chakra that typically deals with this condition. My philosophy is to start with simple treatments. If that simple treatment does not work, then more complex treatments become necessary. The Sacral chakra Key points of Gov 12 and PC 3 were needled and stimulated every five minutes. Next the Sacral chakra acupoint of Con 6 and the Throat chakra point Con 22 (coupled chakra) were needled. Finally the Source points of the associated meridians, Spleen and Pericardium—SP 3 and PC 7, were needled. Debbie was advised to rest for the remainder of the day. A future appointment was made for the following week.

SECOND TREATMENT SESSION

Debbie returned saying that she had felt better but noted that the hot flashes had only improved marginally. I decided in her second session to introduce the eight extraordinary meridians combined with chakra acupuncture to attempt to improve the production of estrogen. I stimulated Bladder 1 (Debbie had given me permission), followed by stimulating the Key points of the *Yinchiao Mai* and *Ren Mai*—KID 6 and LU 7. Then I stimulated the special points Con 4 and Con 7, the Key points of the Sacral chakra—PC 3 and Gov 12, and needled the Sacral chakra acupoint Con 6. Gov 12 was merely stimulated and withdrawn due to its position on the spine. The remaining points were *in situ* for the entire treatment time to enable Debbie to stay in the supine position. She almost fell asleep during the session.

THIRD TREATMENT SESSION

Debbie returned one week later to inform me that she had had a much better week and had only experienced two mild hot flashes. I decided to repeat the previous treatment and advised her to telephone me the next week. She contacted me with the news that she had been "flash free" and was feeling relieved. She did not require any further treatment and was discharged feeling very happy and telling all her friends.

Cervical Spondylosis

James was a sixty-year-old laboratory technician who had suffered from cervical spondylosis for ten years. He had tried TCM acupuncture as well as osteopathy, physical therapy and reflexology. He took codeine and acetaminophen (Tylenol) two or three times a day and the occasional diclofenac if the pain became too severe. He was becoming tolerant of these drugs. Decompression surgery had been ruled out as the MRI had shown there was no focal point for surgery to be successful.

HISTORY AND SYMPTOMS

James had been born with a mid-thoracic scoliosis and had been told that the neck had become arthritic due to the misalignment of the spine as well as his long-term poor posture in his work. The mid-thoracic scoliosis had become arthritic and was causing as much discomfort as the neck. The neck had become increasingly worse over the previous five years and he was forced to wear a soft support collar while working. He suffered from generalized paresthesia in the shoulders and arms, burning neck pain, a feeling of constant pressure in his head, and constant dizziness. His legs felt "heavy" and walking was often a problem. He had suffered from severe indigestion which was corrected by hiatus hernia surgery. From the examination, I decided to balance the Base chakra (chronic and bone-related conditions) as well as to ease the neck pain with minor chakra treatment.

FIRST TREATMENT SESSION

There was sufficient time following the consultation to treat or balance the Base chakra. I explained to James that I would not be working on the neck initially but that the basis or "foundation" of his problem needed to be addressed. The Base chakra Key points Con 22 and LR 8 were stimulated initially and every five minutes during the twenty minutes that the needles were *in situ.* The chakra acupoints of both Gov 2 and Con 2 were needled (he was on his side), followed by needling the Crown chakra (couple) acupoint at Gov 20. The treatment was reinforced by stimulating the Source points of the associated meridians (Kidney and Bladder) at KID 3 and BL 64. He was told to relax as much as he could.

SECOND TREATMENT SESSION

James reported that he had slept "like a baby" the night of the treatment and that during the week he had felt better about himself—a sensation of inner-strength. I decided to treat the cervical and thoracic region with the minor chakras. The cervical region is governed by Schedule One. The mid-thoracic region is governed by Schedule Five. These two regions were treated at the same time. The Key points of Schedules One and Five— HT 6, KID 3, TE 4, and GB 37 were needled and stimulated every five minutes. The chakra acupoints—KID 1, PC 8, TE 17, and SP 21 were needled and left alone *in situ*. James was surprised that I had not placed any needles in the neck or thoracic region.

THIRD TREATMENT SESSION

James returned one week later informing me that the pain in the neck had lessened but that the thoracic pain had worsened. He had started wearing his collar less often. I explained the naturopathic principle to him that states that healing works from inside to outside and that symptoms appear in reverse order from which they came originally. After that, James accepted readily that he was healing himself according to naturopathic principles and agreed to repeat the treatment. We made another appointment for two weeks later.

FOURTH TREATMENT SESSION

James reported that the neck and mid-spine felt much better and that he had discarded his soft collar. The heavy-headed feeling and dizziness were better but were still apparent, and the indigestion had returned. Examination of the abdomen, tongue, and pulse indicated that the Solar Plexus chakra was in a state of imbalance. I intimated to him that we had merely "peeled back some of the layers of the onion" and that he had probably been born with an imbalance in this chakra due to the thoracic scoliosis.

The Key points Con 17 and TE 4 were needled and stimulated every five minutes. Subsequently I needled the chakra points Con 12 and Gov 6 (I decided to treat both anterior and posterior aspects of the Solar plexus chakra due to the symptoms). Third I sedated the coupled Heart chakra at Con 17. The treatment was reinforced by the Source points of the Liver and Stomach meridians—LR 3 and ST 42. Although he was relaxed, it was obvious that he was becoming a little emotional during the session and had a good cry when he sat up. He telephoned me a few days later to tell me that he felt better than he had in years. James came back to see me three months later for a check-up.

CHRONIC DEPRESSION

David was just seventeen years old when he first consulted me. I had previously treated his mother with chronic catarrh and had intimated to her that acupuncture could help with emotional imbalances as well as physical ones. Although slightly reluctant to submit to "alternative" medical treatment and secretive about his problem he was very cooperative in his dialogue with his mother (who had accompanied him) and with me.

HISTORY AND SYMPTOMS

David's birth had been difficult. He was born with the cord around the neck and had required resuscitation to survive. His mother described him as a "morose" child who had been reluctant to play with other children. Rather than the popular music his peers enjoyed, he preferred classical music and art and was decidedly a loner. He was very aware of his illness and his shortcomings and would have given anything to be like the other kids. He was lean and wiry and was not interested in food. He had attended regular psychotherapy as a teenager, which mostly used cognitive approaches. David did not feel he had benefited from psychotherapy. He had also taken many different prescription drugs with little to no effect. Unlike many of my younger patients he was unafraid of needles so we decided to try an acupuncture treatment. Analysis of the abdomen, tongue, and pulse indicated that the Heart and Solar Plexus chakras needed help.

FIRST TREATMENT SESSION

The Heart chakra and the Solar Plexus chakra are coupled so there are fewer points to treat than with disparate chakras. The Key points of the Heart chakra and Solar Plexus—Gov 7, HT 1, Con 17, and TE 4—were inserted and stimulated every five minutes. I needled the chakra point of the Solar Plexus Con 12 (remember the Heart meridian acupoint is the same as the Key point of the Solar Plexus chakra). Finally I needled the Source points of the associated meridians of Heart, Small Intestine, Liver, and Stomach—HT 7, SI 4, LR 3, and ST 42. He was quite weary by the end of the session and was advised to rest.

SECOND TREATMENT SESSION

Although I was not meant to see him for a week, he called two days after his first session to ask if he could be treated again sooner. He reported that he had felt better inside and had felt "lighter." He wanted to keep the momentum going. My analysis indicated that the Solar Plexus chakra seemed to be balanced, so I decided to treat him with the Heart, Ear, and Intercostal combination because of the chronicity of the condition. The Key points Gov 7, HT 1, TE 4, and GB 37 were needled and stimulated every five minutes. This was followed by needling the chakra points Con 17, TE 17, and SP 21. The Source points of the Spleen and Triple Energizer meridians were not required. I told him to come back in one week.

THIRD TREATMENT SESSION

David had felt very good about himself but was having a recurring nightmare about feeling strangled. I read his nightmare as a sign that his body was reacting to his birth trauma, the root of his emotional troubles. He was very happy to receive further treatment. Because the initial shock to his psyche was the cause of his emotional disorder, I decided to balance the Crown chakra. The Key points Con 4 and TE 5 were needled and stimulated every five minutes. Then I needled the chakra point Gov 20. During this third session I decided to hold his heels in order "ground" him. At the end of the treatment he was extremely relaxed and admitted that his brain felt as if "there was fresh air in it"—and could he please come again!

FOURTH TREATMENT SESSION

David was off all psychiatric medication by his fourth treatment and, according to his parents, was a different young man than the few weeks prior. His exhibit of positive behavior was very encouraging but I warned his parents against complacency. I decided to repeat the previous treatment. He came to see me once a month for several months to maintain his emotional stability.

The above Case Histories represent a cross section of the hundreds of patients who have been treated using this type of acupuncture. Please do not be tempted by adding different acupoints during the treatment session. I know it is hard not to add a couple of the tried and tested TCM points for certain conditions. I have found that the extra points merely negate the intended result. Stick to the methods that I have given to you. You will not be disappointed.

APPENDIX ONE—
COPPER AND ZINC NEEDLES

THE USE OF COPPER AND ZINC NEEDLES
WITH THE CHAKRA ENERGY SYSTEM

I have used copper and zinc needles for over thirty years in clinical practice. They make a wonderful alternative to ordinary stainless steel needles and are ideal for use with subtle energies. Naturally they may also be considered in non-chakra acupuncture. These two metals have opposite magnetic affects. Copper is used predominantly in acute and *yang* conditions. Zinc is used predominantly in chronic and *yin* conditions. Because these needles have opposite magnetic polarities, are extremely fine, and barely pierce the outer layer of the epidermis, they are admirably suited to chakra acupuncture. These small needles work with Etheric energies and not those of the Physical Body. There are advantages and disadvantages to picking copper and zinc needles over stainless steel needles.

ADVANTAGES

• They need not, strictly, be pre-sterilized as they do not actually pierce the skin and would never draw blood. Hygiene, though, would dictate that they be kept in a sterilizing solution, e.g., chlorhexidine (hibitane).

• Because copper and zinc possess opposite magnetic polarities, they are ideally suited to energy balancing.

• Copper and zinc needles may be used by non-professional acupuncturists for the reasons stated above.

- Copper and zinc needles have an advantage over stainless steel needles in the treatment of many emotional conditions such as anxiety and stress.
- The treatment of children and of patients with needle phobia is particularly appropriate with copper and zinc needles which are less invasive.

DISADVANTAGES

- The needles are minuscule—total length just over half an inch (one centimeter)—so they are often tricky to pick up and place *in situ.*
- Because of their size, they are easily lost especially if placed on a *hirsute* area of the body. They need to be "counted out and counted back" when placed and removed.
- Because they do not penetrate the skin and therefore do not affect the acupoint as such, they are not recommended in generalized acupuncture treatments.
- For their size, they are relatively expensive.
- As they say, you pay your money and take your choice. Needles are a personal preference.

TECHNIQUES

The following represent some of the options that are open to you when using the chakra energy approach with these needles:

1. When treating an individual chakra, major or minor, place the zinc needles "on" (not "in" as the skin is not pierced) the Key point or points and the copper needle on the chakra point. There is no need to stimulate the Key point.

2. When balancing a chakra with its coupled chakra, make sure that the copper needle is placed on the chakra to be treated and the zinc needle placed on the couple to achieve a magnetic balance.

3. These needles are sometimes successful in the pain relief for-mula with the minor chakras, especially when treating children (see Chapter Three). They are not, however, a treatment of choice. Once again make sure that the zinc needles are placed on the Key points and the copper ones on the chakra points.

4. If required these needles may be placed on the foot reflected chakras (see my book *Healing with the Chakra Energy System* for placement). This makes a perfect adjunct approach for the reflexologist. It also is a great treatment protocol for patients who do not like to be needled or touched anywhere on the body (these people exist).

5. These needles are very useful when used in conjunction with stainless steel needles in general acupuncture work. For exam-ple copper and zinc needles are useful when used with stainless steel needles in the treatment of shingles. The pain relief sched-ule uses stainless steel needles while copper needles are placed around the shingles region, approximately one inch apart and in a complete circle. With subsequent treatment sessions the shingles area (and the pain) narrows so fewer copper needles are required. Another example is with the treatment of scar tis-sue. The scarring can be anywhere on the body but may have proved problematic with other approaches, e.g., ultrasound or deep massage. Scar tissue often blocks the natural flow of energy, blood, and lymph. It is imperative that its pliability is improved. Zinc needles are placed completely around the scar tissue at approximately half an inch distant from each other. It is help-ful if they are placed around scarring following the application of silica ointment that has been previously massaged into the area. The localized treatment of Dupuytren's contracture answers very well to this approach.

APPENDIX TWO—
BIOMAGNETICS

BIOMAGNETIC THERAPY AND THE CHAKRAS

Magnets of all kinds have been used in healing for many centuries. According to legend, the properties of the magnet have been known since the day when they were accidentally discovered by Magnes, a Greek shepherd. He was taking his sheep to pasture, passed a large rock, and found his iron-mounted staff being pulled toward it by an unknown force. He had to exert all his strength to tear it away. The rock was named the Magnet Stone. It is said that being amazed by the force and wishing to make use of it, he inserted pieces of the stone inside his sandals which enabled him to cover longer distances at one stretch without getting tired. The story of Magnes may only be a myth, but in it there is a grain of truth.

It is known that there are natural magnetic forces in and around the earth. There is lodestone in the earth and the earth itself has a magnetic field which is scientifically measurable. We also know that the moon has a magnetic pull on the earth which is so powerful that it affects the oceans of the world. It also has the power to affect the water content within humans and animals (as well as plants). There has been much research carried out regarding the weight of vegetables and plants changing in relation to the various phases of the moon. Scientists have proven that the average human being weighs a few ounces more during the full moon of the lunar cycle and less at the new moon of the lunar cycle. Scientists have proven that the human body is a source of magnetism and measurement of the ion currents of the heart and brain have been carried out by magnetocardiogram and magnetoencephalogram—see *The Book of Magnetic Healing* by Roger Coghill, published by Gaia Books (2000). The human body is also a receiver for incoming electromagnetic energies. Magnetism seems to affect every cell in the physical body as well as the aura. The magnetic field seems to exert an influence on diencephalon which controls the endocrine system. It is known that the endocrine system has a powerful influence on the body's hormonal chemistry and that the chakras influence the endocrine glands. Thus, it makes sense that by positioning magnets on the body at the correct places, the body's magnetism and hormonal chemistry can be influenced.

There has been resurgence in the use of magnets over the past few years as being genuine alternatives to "suppressive" forms of medicine. One can now acquire magnetic necklaces, bracelets, cervical collars, insoles, belts, cushions, pads, and blankets, as well as individual magnets. Magnetic therapy is included within the whole field of energy medicine as being a tool to bring about harmony of the individual part as well as the whole. There are many different types of magnets, each with different strengths (measured in gauss) and actions.

There appears, however, to be confusion in the world of magnetics as to magnets use in healing. Many years ago magnets were used (often powered by a mini-generator) to encourage the healing of bone fractures that had not mended using other procedures. These particular magnets were of enormous strength in the order of two thousand gauss. Since those days it has been found that subtle use of magnets works best and the gauss strength of the ordinary magnet used in, say, a bracelet is in the range of three to four gauss. This strength is enormously different compared to the strength of the super magnets that were once used.

The original concept of Biomagnetic therapy was introduced to the Western world about thirty years ago by Dr. Osamu Itoh of Japan. Research and subsequent teaching in the field of Biomagnetics continued through the work of the British Biomagnetic Association, headed by Dr. Terence Williams of Torquay, Devon. This Association still exists and is located at the Williams Clinic at 31 St. Marychurch Road, Torquay, UK, although its founder passed on several years ago.

When I first learned how to use Biomagnetic therapy, the magnets were placed on the Key points or Command points of the eight extraordinary meridians which achieved positive results on the whole in the field of hormonal energy balancing. When my interest in using the subtle energies in healing took over I decided to experiment with them on the chakras. One of the main differences between biomagnets and other types is that the magnetic strength of each magnet is very low at four-tenths of one gauss. This magnetic force is comparable with the human body's own subtle energy magnetic strength. This is what makes the magnets so effective —the strength is correct and the points used are correct. There are two polarities to a biomagnet. The white colored biomagnets are south pole or positive. The green colored biomagnets are north pole or negative. The magnets are tiny and can become easily lost. Each biomagnet is approximately one-fifth of an inch (four millimeters) in diameter while the actual magnet which is embedded in the center on the underside is just one-twentieth of an inch (one millimeter) in diameter.

Here is a list of the uses of biomagnets:

• Biomagnets are popular with patients who do not like the invasive approaches of acupuncture.
• Children especially like Biomagnetic therapy which does not involve needles.
• Conditions that answer well to Biomagnetic therapy with the chakras are those that involve hormonal imbalance, the general chemistry of the body, and the more subtle energy imbalances.
• Stress-related conditions answer well to approaches using biomagnets, as does the treatment of headaches.
• Treatments may be enhanced by combining the therapy with either acupuncture or reflexology. Never be afraid to mix and match with the individual therapies.

Biomagnets are easy to apply with good quality sticky tape. Patients must be warned, however, when they are removed, especially in *hirsute* areas.

TREATMENT OF THE MAJOR CHAKRAS USING BIOMAGNETIC THERAPY

Treatment of the individual chakras uses the same points as are used in acupuncture and acupressure. The golden rule is that green magnets (negative) are placed on the chakra points and white magnets (positive) are placed on the Key points. More than one chakra may be treated at the same time although it is not a practical proposition to treat more than two at any time. The magnets are left *in situ* for about twenty minutes while the patient lies down relaxing or receiving other therapies such as acupuncture or reflexology (so long as the same points are not required). Patients must be kept warm and relaxed, so it is best to let them rest.

ENERGY BALANCING THE MINOR CHAKRAS USING BIOMAGNETIC THERAPY

One of the simplest ways to balance the patient's vital force is to place magnets on the minor chakras. This is a method I often use when patients visit who have no particular problem or condition *but want to stay well*. It is a simple, non-invasive method. The patient may nod off a couple of minutes after the treatment begins and wake-up refreshed at the end of half an hour or so. All twenty minor chakras (not the Spleen chakra) are balanced. Green magnets are placed on one minor chakra and the white magnets are placed on the coupled chakra. This needs to be done bilaterally.

White (positive) magnets are placed on:
- Hand chakra at PC 8
- Elbow chakra at PC 3
- Shoulder chakra at LI 15
- Ear chakra at TE 17
- Clavicular chakra at KID 27

Green (negative) magnets are placed on:
- Foot chakra at KID 1
- Knee chakra at BL 40
- Groin chakra at ST 30

- Intercostal chakra at SP 21
- Navel chakra at KID 16

TREATMENT OF THE MINOR CHAKRAS USING BIOMAGNETIC THERAPY

Low gauss biomagnets are very useful in the treatment of pain in association with the minor chakras. Acute and semi-acute pain answers to magnet treatment very well, but chronic pain needs the deeper approach that acupuncture can offer. The rule of thumb is always to place the green magnet (north pole—negative) on the chakra points and the white magnets (south pole—positive) on the Key points. Therefore a magnetic balance is created between the chakra and its Key point. An example of this type of treatment would be for hand pain, where you would use Schedule 1 and place the green magnets on PC 8 and KID 1 and the white magnets on KID 3 and HT 6. These points are inserted bilaterally and left *in situ* for about twenty minutes or until the discomfort eases. More than one Schedule may be treated at a time although it is rare to treat more than two. If warranted the associated meridians may be stroked using acupressure to enhance the treatment.

TREATMENT OF COMBINATION OF MAJOR AND MINOR CHAKRAS USING BIOMAGNETICS

As previously stated, the conditions that react favorably to Biomagnetic therapy are acute pain, hormonal imbalance, and those associated with stress, e.g., anxiety, palpitations, stress-triggered migraine, etc. Below are five of the six chakra combinations (as described in Chapter One) listed with a typical condition and Biomagnetic treatment for your reference.

1. CROWN, HAND, AND FOOT COMBINATION

Suggested Condition: Stress-related Migraine

A stress-related migraine is a condition that answers extremely well to this approach in that the *cause* is being addressed. By using the subtlety of magnets, a shift in the patient's energy pattern will begin to control the migraine as well as relieving other symptoms such as tense neck, tense stomach muscles, and acidic stomach. Subsidiary treatment with reflexology may also be required.

Method—Place the green (north pole) magnets on the chakra points of GOV 20, PC 8, and KID 1 and the white magnets (south pole) on the Key points of CON 4, TE 5, KID 3, and HT 6. The magnets stay *in situ* for between twenty to thirty minutes. Remember to keep the patient warm, this really does help—do not be stingy with the warm towels. There is nothing worse for a patient than to have to lie still for a length of time feeling cold—it defeats the object of treatment.

2. BROW, GROIN, AND CLAVICULAR COMBINATION

Suggested Condition: Bottled-up Rage and Anger

While being symptomatic of a cause outside the healing potential of the therapist, the treatment suggested affects the subtle energies enough to strengthen the patient and their resolve to come to terms with the true cause. This routine surely has to be preferable to taking tranquilizers and other mind-affecting drugs.

- *Method*—Place the green magnets on the chakra points GOV 16, Extra 1 *(Yintang)*, ST 30, and KID 27 and the white magnets on the Key points GOV 4, SP 6, LR 8, and PC 7.

3. THROAT, SHOULDER, AND NAVEL COMBINATION

Suggested Condition: Shyness

Shyness could either be temporary or a more permanent form of introversion. Shyness treatment can also be used for someone unable to express themselves or suffering from inability to think clearly ("brain fog").

- *Method*—Place the green magnets on the chakra points of CON 22, GOV 16, LI 15, and KID 16 and place the white magnets on the Key points of CON 6, LR 5, ST 40, and LI 11.

4. HEART, EAR, AND INTERCOSTAL COMBINATION

Suggested Condition: Grief or Tearfulness

The Heart, Ear and Intercostal combination is the one most used in Biomagnetic therapy, because it may be used in various different circumstances. Countless people from a jilted groom to a mourning widow have harbored grief for months or even years and may have formed a block to further treatment. Every day we meet patients who appear to be tearful for some reason. This approach will help them to resolve the situation—keep the tissues handy!

- *Method*—Place the green magnets on the chakra points of CON 17, GOV 10, TE 17, and SP 21 and place the white magnets on the Key points of GOV 7, HT 1, TE 4, and GB 37.

5. SACRAL, SOLAR PLEXUS, AND SPLEEN COMBINATION

Suggested Condition: Pre-menstrual Tension

Pre-menstrual tension is just one of the gynecological symptom pictures that may be addressed with this combination. Others include dysmenorrhea and hot flashes.

- *Method*—Place the green magnets on the chakra points of GOV 3, CON 6, GOV 6, CON 12, and SP 16 and place the white magnets on the Key points of CON 17, TE 4, GOV 12, PC 3, and GOV 8

Unfortunately, the sixth combination of Base, Elbow, and Knee does not work with biomagnets because the Base chakra is used predominantly to treat chronic conditions. The Elbow and Knee chakras may be used singly or in combination to treat painful conditions associated with these minor chakras.

Please note that there are many other ways of using Biomagnetic therapy than I have delineated here. The methods outlined in this Appendix are for exclusive use with the chakra energy system, but there are many other Biomagnetic methods that can be utilized in other ways than with chakras. Magnets are safe, relatively cheap, non-invasive, and very effective. They are a worthy investment, and I urge you to try to use them to help your patients.

REFERENCES

Academy of Traditional Chinese Medicine. *An Outline of Chinese Acupuncture.* Beijing: Foreign Language Press, 1975.

Brennan, B.A. *Hands of Light: A Guide to Healing Through the Human Energy Field.* New York: Bantam, 1987.

Coghill, R. *The Book of Magnetic Healing.* London: Gaia Books, 2000.

Cross, J.R. *Acupressure: Clinical Applications in Musculo-Skeletal Conditions.* Oxford, England: Butterworth Heinemann, 2000.

———. *Acupressure and Reflextherapy in Medical Conditions,* Oxford, England: Butterworth Heinemann, 2001.

———. *Healing with the Chakra Energy System—Acupressure, Bodywork and Reflexology for Total Health.* Berkeley: North Atlantic Books, 2006.

———. "The Relationship of the Chakra Energy System and Acupuncture." PhD diss., British College of Acupuncture, 1986.

Gerber, R. *Vibrational Medicine—New Choices for Healing Ourselves.* Santa Fe: Bear and Company, 1988.

Leadbeater, C.W. *The Chakras.* 1927. Reprint, Wheaton, IL: Theosophical Publishing House, 1982.

McNaught, A., and R. Callender. *Illustrated Physiology.* London: E and S Livingstone, 1965.

Motoyama, H. *Theory of the Chakras: Bridge to Higher Consciousness.* Wheaton: Theosophical Publishing House, 1988.

Myers T.W. *Anatomy Trains—Myofascial Meridians for Manual and Movement Therapists.* Oxford, England: Churchill Livingstone, 2001.

Oschman, J.L. *Energy Medicine—The Scientific Basis.* Edinburgh, Scotland: Churchill Livingstone, 2000.

————. *Energy Medicine in Therapeutics and Human Performance.* Oxford, England: Butterworth Heinemann, 2003.

Tansley, D.V. *Radionics and the Subtle Anatomy of Man.* Cambridge, England: C.W. Daniel, 1972.

Williams, T. *Complete Chinese Medicine: A Comprehensive System for Health and Fitness.* Bath, England: Element Books, 1996.

Young, J. *The Healing Path: The Practical Guide to the Holistic Traditions of China, India, Tibet and Japan.* Wellingborough, England: Thorsons, 2001.

Zong-Xiang, Z. "Research Advances in the Electrical Specificity of Meridians and Acupuncture Points." *American Journal of Acupuncture* 9, no. 3 (1981): 203–17.

INDEX